# TRIUMPH OVER ILLNESS

## Dr. WILLIAM S. GANDEE

**Avery Publishing Group**
Garden City Park, New York

The publisher does not advocate the use of any particular form of health care but believes the information presented in the book should be available to the public. The information and procedures contained in this book are based upon the research and personal and professional experiences of the author. They are not intended as a substitute for consulting with your health-care provider. The publisher and author are not responsible for any adverse effects or consequences resulting from the use of any suggestions or procedures discussed in this book. All matters pertaining to your physical health should be supervised by a health-care professional.

Cover Design: Timothy Boylan
Typesetting: Al Berotti
In-House Editor: Dara Stewart


**Avery Publishing Group**
120 Old Broadway
Garden City Park, NY 11040
1-800-548-5757

Library of Congress Cataloging-in-Publication Data

Gandee, William S.
    Triumph over illness: what you should know about the power of chiropractic care/ William S. Gandee, Peggy Russell.
    p. cm.
    Includes index.
    ISBN 0-89529-818-X
    1. Chiropractic—Popular works. I. Russell, Peggy. II. Title.
    RZ241.G36 1997
    615.5'34—dc21                                                      97-34719
                                                                            CIP

Printed in the United States of America

10  9  8  7  6  5  4  3  2  1

# Contents

*Chapter*

The role of the health-care provider—whether a doctor of traditional medicine or of an alternate form of health care—should always be to serve the best interest of the patient. This chapter will discuss how some traditional medicine and chiropractic care can, and should, work together, in the best interest of the patient.

This chapter discusses the history of chiropractic care— where it began, and what it does and doesn't do.

Some people don't know what to expect on their first visit to a chiropractor. Who are these health care professionals? What are they like? What happens when we step into a chiropractor's office?

Many people think a "bad back" is the only reason to go to a chiropractor. Even if that were true, let's examine how very important the back can be to your overall good health and well-being.

What a magnificent creation you are! Your body was designed to keep you from harm's way. It is only when we tamper with that original design that our bodies begin to experience difficulty in running in top form.

# Acknowledgements

It seems as if I have been writing this book my entire life, and if the truth be told—I have been for most of it. There have been many who have contributed to this book's content—some with the love that they have given me, some with the effect they've had on my life, and others due to their thoughts, ideas, and the path that they have helped me seek. As one of my favorite motivational speakers Charles "Tremendous" Jones once said, "The only difference in yourself between now and in five years are the people you meet and the books you read."

My parents, Bill and Louise Gandee, have always stood behind me in whatever I've done. They provided me with a good, moral, Christian childhood. I couldn't have had better parents. My wife, Debbie, and my two children, Steven and Lauren, are among the true pleasures of my life. My entire family—grandparents, aunts, uncles, cousins, and especially my sister Donna—has supported chiropractic even though they initially did not understand it.

The founder of Life Chiropractic College, Dr. Sid Williams, and his wife, Nell, must be thanked for their vision, their determination and their success. Life Chiropractic College has grown and is now Life University. Their story is truly one of success against impossible odds.

My favorite professor at Life Chiropractic College was Gerald Clum. He was truly an inspiration. There is not a mean bone in his body. He is a great man in chiropractic, and the good of our profession is foremost in his heart.

I must thank my two best friends, Dr. Rick Franks and Dr. John Kelly. We spent many hours brainstorming about chiropractic philosophy, ideology, and procedures. Together, we are one.

In my own office, I continue to see daily the wonders of chiropractic. I still enjoy seeing new patients discover its "secrets" and then shout it from the rooftops to all who will listen. My patients, past, present, and future, are the real reason that I've written this book. It is to them that I owe a great debt of gratitude, love, and thanks.

Over the years I've been blessed with great people who work with me in my professional office. My staff, most of whom have worked with me for years, helped keep me focused, grounded, and able to concentrate on helping people. They took care of the office, and they made my life so much easier. Thank you all.

I would like to thank my agent, Frank Weimann, for his enormous help in finding the right publisher at the right time. I can only hope that this is the beginning of a long, multifaceted relationship.

At Avery Publishing, I must remember those who have offered their expertise, time, and knowledge in making this book a reality. I must especially thank Rudy Shur for his guidance and Dara Stewart who did the final editing with great professional finesse, dedication, and patience.

Then there is Peggy Russell. Peggy has struggled through every word and sentence of this book, trying to decipher the logic behind my writing. She did more research than you could imagine. I could not have written this book without her. She is a unique person. She is strong in opinion, yet compassionate in discussion. There aren't many Peggy Russells in the world.

Last, but not least, I would like to thank my God and savior Jesus Christ. In Him all things are possible. And if it is His will, I ask that this book open millions of people's eyes to the concept of true health, alternative health—chiropractic health.

# Introduction

I love people. I know, you hear that a lot, but I really do love people. I believe I have shown this to be true by dedicating my life to the good health of those with whom I come in contact. My sincere love of people is the primary reason for writing this book. That fact will become clear to you as you continue to read.

My heart breaks when I see so much pain, sickness, and unnecessary suffering. It is even worse knowing that there is *a better way*, and that many people either do not know, or do not understand, the concept of good health. They do not know, as I do, that good chiropractic care, natural health, and common sense have the answers many people seek all their lives. I hope that this book can open some eyes, get some "amens," and show that there is indeed a better way of life . . . and health.

The saddest part of the untold health story, I believe, is that the health care system, as it is known today, has sold everybody out. We've been sold out for a lot more than thirty pieces of silver. I am talking billions of dollars here. Those who profit from what I can't help but call "the big lie" do not want you to be healthy. They do not want you to be educated about your health. They want you to be sick and under their control. They want you dependent on them for help. Even more abominable is the fact that those who are aware of "the big lie" continue to teach it as truth to those who are honestly in search of a way to help humankind through medical means and believe—as they have been taught—that this is the only way.

For many years we have accepted sickness, disease, and slow, painful death as a way of life. It is considered "normal." We are taught to believe sickness and pain are the natural paths our lives take. Can we honestly believe that God wants us to be ill, that He gave us weak and inept bodies that fall apart by the age of 30 or 40? We've bought the lie that tells us that in order to be healthy, we need to take drugs so our bodies can continue to function the "natural" way. Once the drugs don't work anymore—and that time usually comes—then we can resort to surgery. If we have a problem body part, we'll simply let the physician take it out and throw it away, and we are as good as new. Well, this is hardly the case.

We continue to allow this to happen every day, if not to our own bodies, then to those we love and cherish. We also allow "the big lie" to continue, and we die long before our allotted time, believing that we've done all we can to be healthy.

"Well, I went to the doctor . . . "

"I did what I was told . . . "

"I took my medicine . . . "

"I had the surgery . . . "

"I said, 'yes, doctor'. . . "

Is that what life is all about? Could there really be a better way? There are some people who know there is, and those of us who do know have a moral responsibility to let others know some of the real truths that we have learned first-hand.

In one Harrison Ford movie, the hero said that being silent is another way of accepting what is said as the truth, and I believe this is an adequate description of what I'm trying to project in this book. Anyone who knows me or who has been a patient of mine knows, without question, that "being silent" is not part of my make-up. For over fifteen years, I've given weekly health talks in my office. I constantly strive to educate my patients and all with whom I come in contact. In addition, I've given numerous health talks outside of my office—in my own communtiy and in other states, as well. Slowly, I am beginning to see an awakening among those I meet on a day-to-day basis. They are beginning to question things they once took as gospel from their family physicians. They are beginning to realize that medicine is not working. If it were, we'd certainly all be in excellent health, considering the amount of money we spend on medicine and the continuing growth of medical facilities around the world. They are also beginning to realize that surgery is not always the answer. They know there is a better way, even before they realize what the better way is. They are opening their minds and their hearts to search for—and find— real, true, and natural answers to good health.

For years we've all heard about the political "silent majority." Just as the voters need to express their opinions that "all is not right" at the polls and something different has to be done, we can expect more of this in our everyday lives as well, particularly when it comes to control of our health. We are tired of letting others make life and death decisions for us, and I truly believe we are seeing the dawn of a new health day.

It's a concept whose time has come. Actually, it's long overdue! If I'd written this book ten or fifteen years ago—maybe even three years ago—the average American might not have been ready to hear or heed its message. I believe the time is finally right for this project. It is my fervent hope that those who read it will tell others about the better way of health that I discuss on these pages. I want you to read the words thoroughly and intently, and then ask yourself these questions about the message this book conveys: Is it logical? Does it make sense? Can I use it? Is it a better way of health care?

I want those of you who are reading these pages to know that I have written this book with love. It is my hope and my earnest prayer that you will read it and use the information to help yourself and your loved ones. Many of you may never have read or heard much of what is written here, but I can tell you that the concepts written on these pages contain the principles of life and health that I've been talking about for fifteen years in my health lectures. In every one of my sessions, I try to emphasize the importance of taking control of your own bodies and charting your own good health care. I am constantly reemphasizing what chiropractors began teaching 100 years ago about the underlying cause of sickness and dis-ease and the underlying reasons for good health and long life, as they are the same today.

If you care about your good health and the good health of those around you, this book is for you. I believe you already know that. That is why you picked it up in the first place, and that is why you will continue to read the words that I've put here for you.

# Chapter 1

# Do No Harm

*One day while out for a walk by a beautiful free-flowing river, a young man happened to notice something floating near the surface. He was horrified to discover, upon closer inspection, that it was a person. Quickly, and without thought of his own life, he jumped into the moving waters. With much effort he rescued the seemingly lifeless body from an almost certain death. Then, using every method of resuscitation he knew of, he set about to revive the helpless victim. After what seemed like an eternity, he detected a faint heartbeat. He was elated. However, no sooner than he had finished his awesome task did he see another body floating downstream, followed closely by two or three more.*

*"I must get help," he thought. "Lots of help."*

*He could not let those people continue to float downstream to their deaths. Soon, a growing group was working diligently to save the helpless people. They enlisted builders who erected a huge structure on the river bank in which to resuscitate the drowning victims.*

*Alas, it was soon filled to capacity. More and more people came to help, but they were always short-handed and overworked, and the flow of victims never let up. They rejoiced over the ones rescued, and mourned over the ones lost.*

*Soon, another young man happened to walk down the river path. He stood for a moment, watching their frantic efforts.*

*"Hey," someone called to him. "Lend us a hand."*

*The young man asked what they were doing.*

*"What does it look like we're doing?" one particularly disgruntled man answered.*

"We're saving lives here. Can't you see that?"

"Yes, I can," he answered politely.

"Then, for God's sake, help us."

"Could I ask a question first?"

"Make it quick," came the answer. "Time is a matter of life and death here!"

"Yes, I can see that as well," he answered. "I admire your work, but . . . " he hesitated, then continued. "Why don't you try to find out why all these people ended up in the water in the first place?"

"Try to find out why?" one gruff voice repeated, as he pulled in two more victims from the swirling waters. "We don't have time to find out why . . . we're too busy trying to save lives."

People are sick . . . and getting sicker. Just look around. You know it's true. We must try to find out why. We should be looking for the cause, not trying to find treatments for the myriad of different symptoms. People are suffering and dying, and we don't know *why!*

Are we asking the right questions? I don't think so.

Motivational speaker Anthony Robbins said if you want better answers, ask better questions. We need to offer people something to make them feel better, something to help them to become—and continue to stay—healthy and well. We need to ask questions concerning what to do, what not to do, or what to change to keep people from getting sick in the first place. We cannot continue simply pulling them out of the waters. We have to find out how they got there in the first place and find a way to prevent them from being in harm's way.

Everybody will agree that "prevention" is an excellent answer. We all subscribe to the "ounce of prevention is worth a pound of cure" theory. This means that it is sixteen times more important to *prevent* an illness from happening, than it is to spend years of effort and millions of dollars searching for a cure. Organized medicine does not really understand prevention in the first place and appears to give it too little regard. In the meantime, the person in need may float into the rapids and disappear.

## THE WHOLE PICTURE

"First of all, do no harm."

This was the basic and noble principle on which mainstream medicine was established. Many medical doctors still subscribe to, and live by, these important words written by Hippocrates, the Father of Medicine.

Hippocrates was right on the money with this admonition. Actually, he had a far different concept of medicine than do many who work in the field today, struggling to save as many lives of those floating down the stream of life as possible.

Why are there so *many* in need of help? Because we are paying for sickness. If you pay for an automobile, you get an automobile—so it stands to reason that if you pay for sickness, you get sickness—and plenty of it. What we should be paying for is good health. Sickness should be free—and rare.

What is causing so many people to be in poor health? Are we so busy trying to rescue them that we neither have the time nor the inclination to find out *why* they are sick?

Actually, some of the reasons are known. Researchers work long hours and tiresome days and nights searching for that one missed molecule, diseased cell, malformed gene, or new idea that will provide answers for a cure—or at least a way to alleviate some of the suffering. Like those men at the river bank, medical doctors' hearts and minds are in the right places, and their efforts are much appreciated by those who are rescued from a certain death and given another chance at life. But something is still missing. We are not getting the whole picture.

It is true that they do not have time to find out why so many are floating downstream—because they are too busy trying to save lives by treating the increasing numbers of victims floating down the stream. However, not only are they not able to save everyone floating downstream, there are also many pulled ashore who still perish. Are they killed by exposure? By whatever put them in peril in the first place? By the rescuers themselves? Unfortunately, the answer is *all of the above*. We've all heard that in too many instances, the treatment is worse than the disease. Medicine can, and does, cause other horrible problems for the person seeking relief from an illness.

## A Seldom Discussed Disease

How many times have you heard someone say they are suffering from an *iatrogenic disease*? How often have you heard that so-and-so just died from an iatrogenic disease? It's not something you hear people talking about, mainly because most people have never even heard the word "iatrogenic," yet it is the fastest growing epidemic in this country, killing over three thousand people a week. "How can this be? Why haven't we heard about it?" you ask.

William Boyd, M.D., author of the classic medical text *Boyd's Pathology*, explains it from the viewpoint of a medical doctor: "In the fear of the public, we seek refuge in a mystic word, 'iatrogenic,' trusting that the patient will not consult a medical dictionary and find that 'Iatros' is Greek for 'physician' and 'genic' means 'produced by.' Unfortunately, what is powerful for good may also be potent for evil."

Am I saying that Americans are dying from physician-caused sickness? That's exactly what I'm saying, and although unintentional, it is, nevertheless, a brutal fact of life and death. Now I am not talking only about malpractice or other medical mistakes. I am talking about a disease causing sickness, impairment, disfigurement, or death caused by the practice of what we, the general public, deem to be "accepted medical care."

Some other rather unsettling events that support the iatrogenic character of medicine can be found in the following:

- A month-long doctor's strike in Israel in 1973 brought a chilling report from the Jerusalem Burial Society. The death rate dropped 50 percent that month. The only time it had ever had such a reduction was twenty years before—the last time the doctors had gone on strike.

- In 1976, the medical doctors in Bogota, Colombia went on a fifty-two day strike. *The National Catholic Reporter* cited a 35-percent drop in the death rate of its citizens during that time.

- Also in 1976, the medical doctors went on strike in Los Angeles County to protest malpractice rates. Death rates dropped 18 percent. To further underscore these figures, it was noted that once the doctors went back to work, death rates went back to "normal."

It does not take a genius to figure out from these accounts that when the doctors were not treating patients, less of them died. Mind-boggling? Yes. Could it be because there was less interference with the natural healing system that was designed to work for us?

Noted author and medical doctor Robert Mendelsohn, whose books *Confessions of a Medical Heretic* and *How to Raise a Healthy Child in Spite of Your Doctor* are extremely informative and highly recommended, has this to say about modern medicine: "I believe that more than 90 percent of modern medicine could disappear from the face of the earth—doctor, hospital, drugs, and equipment—and the effect on our health would be immediate and beneficial."

A harsh and shocking condemnation? Perhaps, but sometimes it takes an almost radical stance in order to get the message across. For example, how many of you know that in 1986, the United States Office of Public Health concluded, after an extensive thirteen-year study, that *two-thirds* of the over-the-counter drugs (pain relievers, antacids, etc.) did not fulfill the promoters' claims? Wouldn't you think this would merit the front page, or at least an exposé on one of the popular magazine television shows? Perhaps even a government grant to study the problem? Unfortunately, there seem to be more important topics:

Let's save the cave bats . . .

We'll study cow flatulence . . .

Let's get serious!

## We Interrupt This Program . . .

Imagine, if you will, that you are watching your favorite television program, and a special news bulletin is announced. Dan Rather appears on the screen and tells you that a horrible earthquake in the western part of the United States has killed 10,000 people.

"That's horrible!" you may say.

You bet it is.

Two months later, Dan, or maybe Tom Brokaw this time, appears on your television screen and reports somberly that in the southwestern portion of the country, another quake has claimed another 10,000 people. The country is in shock. Six weeks later,

Peter Jennings interrupts your favorite game show and tells you that yet another quake in the northeastern United States has taken 12,000 more lives. You cannot believe the pain these events must be causing countless numbers of your fellow human beings—or perhaps even your own loved ones who are living in some of these areas. Even if you have no friends or relatives in these regions, your heart cries out for what this terrible disaster has wrought upon the earth. Already 32,000 people have died, and the year is not half over.

There is more bad news. Within the next few months, earthquakes take another 5,000 people in the South, 3,000 in the Southeast, and finally another 12,000 all over the world have been killed in one disaster or another. Some of these casualties include your relatives and loved ones, and you cannot sleep for fear that you may be next. If the newscasters reported that more than 52,000 people had died terrible, and for the most part *preventable*, deaths, within a period of twelve months, we would not even begin to be able to comprehend the horror of it all.

Scary stories? No, these are simple statistics. About earthquakes? No, about the medical profession. Over 1,000 people perish every week (some statistics claim much, *much* higher numbers) just from medication prescribed by the family physician. Arthritis medications *alone* account for more deaths than do heroin, crack cocaine, and all other illegal drugs combined. We are suffering (and dying) from too many drugs, drug reactions, and unnecessary surgery—in general, too much doctoring!

According to *Science Magazine,* 2 to 3 percent of all hospital admissions are primarily due to a negative reaction to drugs. Adding insult to injury, 5 percent of all hospital patients contract new infections after they've been admitted, increasing their hospital stay an average of seven days. In 1980, 1.5 million patients were victims of hospital-acquired infections and about 15,000 of them died. Even the American Medical Association's (AMA's) own journal states that the number of deaths due to hospital-caused mistakes may be equivalent to *"three jumbo jet crashes every two days."* A Boeing 747 jumbo jet carries 452 passengers, so if we use the AMA's figures, this means that 678 people die every day from hospital mistakes, giving us an awesome total of more than 247,000 *preventable* deaths annually. These figures make the 52,000 people a year sound almost insignificant, don't they? But have these numbers made the evening news? Page one of the newspaper? Could you imagine the terror of being told about this carnage on your television screen every other day. *Three more jumbo jets crash—and all 1,356 people aboard are dead!*

I cannot be more graphic than that. Would there be a public outcry to stop the horror of all these airline deaths? Would the deaths of these airline passengers be any more final than the deaths of those who died from physician-caused illness?

Instead, why couldn't we scan the obituaries and read about those who have lived a long and healthy life and died from *natural* causes? "Ninety-Nine-Year-Old Man Dies in His Sleep After Working His Usual Ten-Hour Day on His Farm" should be a headline that we see more often. Dying at a very old age from natural causes is a natural and unavoidable event, and is certainly a preferable way to die. Having one's life cut short by a doctor or medication is, or should be, unacceptable.

Of course, I must also point out that deaths from prescription medicine may sometimes be the fault of the patient who takes too much, takes it incorrectly, or mixes the wrong medicines together due to carelessness, ignorance, or their trying too hard to relieve their pain. Death may also be caused by the wrong prescription or dosage ordered by the doctor, or a fatal mistake made by either the doctor or druggist. Death could be due to any number of reasons, but the end results are the same.

Over 52,000 people a year are dead due to iatrogenic disease and not a single news flash from Tom, Dan, or Peter. The deaths of these people are just as tragic as if they had been swallowed up in an earthquake, caught in a fire, killed in a plane crash, or drowned in a raging flood. The families still grieve, and lives are forever altered in the worst possible ways. The numbers are staggering, yet you haven't heard any of these numbers mentioned in the mainstream media. Why aren't these reports given on the evening news? Even Oprah, Geraldo, *60 Minutes* and *20/20* have failed us—and you thought they'd told us about everything!

## WHO'S WATCHING THE STORE?

The medical profession is in charge of our health because we have been told again and again that "Doctor Knows Best." We continue with what we have, hoping for the best, but usually getting the worst. We cannot assume that the prime concern of organized medicine is our good health. We have to question whether or not we are being deprived of effective and economical health care because those kinds of treatments are not highly profitable for medical doctors, surgeons, and pharmaceutical companies. Unfortunately, we have to consider the facts that support the concept that greed (and even ignorance) sometimes override all moral and humanitarian considerations.

In the book *Racketeering in Medicine—The Suppression of Alternatives* by James P. Carter, M.D., disturbing evidence is presented that bona fide therapies are being disparaged as quackery, health-care givers who offer alternative treatments are being persecuted, government agencies are participating in the harassment of alternative practitioners, drug companies are unduly influencing medical professionals' actions, and kangaroo courts are convicting honorable men and women of trumped-up charges. The financial bottom line all too often determines what types of treatment are researched, tested, and approved.

Dr. Carter states that we must be more aware of health-care practices, and we must speak up for our rights.

The American public has no idea how politics secretly control the practice of medicine. If a doctor dares to introduce a natural, less costly method, no matter how safe or effective, Organized American Medicine can target this doctor for license revocation, using fear tactics and legal maneuvering. Why do holistic therapies threaten medicine? They involve a major change in scientific thought, they imply that current methods are inadequate, and they threaten huge profits of a powerful branch of medicine or a drug company.

Dr. Carter goes on to point out that heart-bypass surgery and balloon angioplasty were quickly embraced and utilized by the medical profession, despite their high risks and costs. While Dr. Carter does not dispute that these new procedures do often

---

# Did You Know...

... that organized medicine describes most holistic approaches as "pseudo-science" and argues that such treatments are "unproven" because double-blind controlled studies have not been performed to prove their efficacy? The fact is that approximately 80 percent of all medical procedures have also never "been proven" through such research studies. Where is the hue and cry over this?

---

save lives as well as improve the quality of life for many, they are basically "money-makers" and were never "proven" by double-blind, placebo-controlled studies, as is required of less risky and cheaper alternative therapies. A Food and Drug Administration (FDA)-required study now costs more than $200 million to complete—which is certainly a deterrent to many serious and brilliant researchers. According to Dr. Carter, "American medicine either doesn't know, or doesn't care about naturally-based medical practices, indigenous to cultures all over the world, that have promoted healing at a fraction of the cost."

Carter's book also details frightening revelations about those who have orchestrated financially motivated cover-ups for the purposes of the following:

- controlling the treatment of heart disease and the related conditions of stroke and peripheral vascular disease.

- controlling the treatment of cancer.

- promoting the use of drugs in the treatment of psychosomatic disorders that respond better to stress management.

- promoting drugs instead of acupuncture to relieve chronic pain.

- discounting natural remedies and nutritional therapies as useless.

- controlling the advancements in the treatment of AIDS, which has remained incurable, in part, because of the failure to consider treatment alternatives.

Hippocrates would be aghast, as you and I should be. The Father of Medicine, I'm sure, would also be very disturbed to see how modern medicine is practiced with an emphasis on drugs and other unnatural chemicals as the choices for treating disease. He would be even more upset to note the ignorance surrounding the importance of nutrition, exercise, and holistic alternative health care. He would certainly not approve of the overuse of surgical procedures and medication in today's medical community. I do not believe that Hippocrates would think that the deaths of more than 52,000 people a year at the hands of the medical community was a result of "doing no harm."

Did Hippocrates believe in chiropractic methods? We have proof in his own writings that he did. Heed the age old wisdom that he left us:

> One or more vertebrae of the spine may or may not go out of place very much. They might give way very little, and, if they do, they are likely to produce serious complications and even death, if not properly adjusted.

He also said, "In all disease, look first to the spine." Could the message be any clearer? Was the Father of Medicine himself advocating spinal adjustments? Of course he was.

## BEST HEALTH CARE MONEY CAN BUY?

Are we spending more money than ever on health care?

The answer is a resounding yes! Americans spent nearly a quarter of a *trillion* dollars in 1986 on health care—twice as much as we spent ten years before, and the numbers climb every year. In 1997, Americans spent over 1 trillion dollars on health care.

Are we now healthier? No.

Is sickness disappearing? On the contrary, it is increasing.

Are we enjoying a healthy old age without being warehoused in a nursing home? No.

Are we taking fewer drugs? Definitely not!

Having fewer surgeries? No! Healthier babies? No!

Enjoying greater peace of mind? No!

Television commercials, radio and newspaper advertisements,

and headlines have given us the impression that everything in the health care field is better than ever. But it is not. Even with the billions of dollars that American medicine is spending on extensive research, modern medical techniques, and the latest diagnostic equipment, we're still very much in pain and in the dark about why so many people are suffering so much. Americans are still sick and still searching for real health answers.

The epidemics of modern civilization—cancer, diabetes, heart disease, mental disorders, hypertension, headaches, allergies, asthma, sinus problems, diverticulitis, ulcers, digestive troubles, ear infections, obesity, sexually transmitted diseases, bacterial infections, and strokes are ravaging us as much as before—and in some cases more then ever. New and more frightening diseases and stronger, meaner, and harder to fight viruses roam like wild animals, seeking to devour their prey.

We are taking *more* pills. (There is an average 800 percent markup on drugs.)

We are having *more* surgery (80 percent of which is believed unnecessary).

We are having *more* tests, *more* procedures, and *more* examinations done. And what do we have? *More* sickness!

And what do we say? "Yes, doctor. Yes, doctor. Yes, doctor!"

We constantly see newspaper stories, television documentaries, and magazine articles that tell of the great breakthroughs in medicine and the wonderful things organized medicine is accomplishing every day. Take your own poll. Check your newspaper for a week, and see how many articles you find *daily* promoting organized medicine. I don't think it would be too harsh to call this blatant propaganda, all designed to manipulate you into believing that the medical profession is your only savior. You will read, every day, about a countless number of new wonder drugs, new types of high-tech surgeries, new methods of testing, new hopes, new dreams, and new goals. Yet we still get the same old results—sickness, disease, and painful, early death.

Medical wonders?

Modern medical miracles?

Better health?

Think about how far we've come—or how far from *natural* remedies we've gone. We have transplants, artificial hearts, and coronary by-pass operations, just to name a few. It is awesome the way our bodies can be altered, dissected, inspected, modified, enhanced, detached, reattached, saved, and, yes, all too often lost in the name of modern medicine.

The optimistic news is that many people are no longer satisfied with answers given by modern medical care. An astounding number of patients are searching for, and finding, better answers. They are beginning to realize, for example, that after years and years and billions of dollars donated to the cancer and heart research funds, these illnesses are still raging, spreading like wildfires, and holding the number one and number two positions as leading causes of deaths.

People are really tired of being sick, and tired of being told they are incapable of making a decision about their own treatment. They want good health, and they want it now. Moreover, they do not want to be harmed in the process by a toxic substance placed in the body that only masks the real problem and does little to correct the underlying cause—and, as a side-effect, may actually kill them.

Hippocrates was a natural healer. He stressed good food, exercise, and various natural remedies, including spinal adjustments, as a means of not only curing diseases but of maintaining good health and preventing further problems.

The term "health-care system" is a misnomer because there is really no such thing in America today. What we have is a "sick-care" system. I can't emphasize enough the fact that we must realize that the real care of a person's health begins *before* sickness, or even *before* the symptoms of sickness set in.

My friends, there is a *better way!* Please read this entire book, and keep an open mind. I believe that education about your health is the pathway to knowledge and wisdom—not to mention peace of mind and just plain old happiness.

Countless studies have been done on the value of chiropractic health care, and each new and conclusive finding supports the belief that this alternative health care system is the preventative care that many have sought for so long.

During World War II, Irvin Hendryson, M.D., a board member of the American Medical Association, did a study of soldiers treated chiropractically and medically. He concluded that the chiropractic techniques were as effective as some of the best

---

### Did You Know...

... that the workers' compensation department of the state of Utah conducted a test in 1986 that showed that chiropractic was ten times more effective than medicine in reducing compensation costs?

---

medical treatments available. In fact, chiropractic had impressive results where conventional medicine failed. He went further to recommend that chiropractic care be an integral part of all army orthopedic wards. His findings were sent to the AMA during the 1940s. And we must give the AMA credit. They did not suppress this study. It was made public . . . *in the 1990s,* some *fifty* years after the study had been done!

## MEDICAL WONDERS

Do I hold that all medical doctors are useless and/or incompetent? Of course not. But do they all fit the Normal Rockwell image? Of course not. There are some aspects about the medical profession that strike awe in many of us. It's amazing, I think, that some have the expertise to perform the quadruple bypass heart surgery. The amount of technical knowledge and skill that goes into these amazing procedures is astounding. My point, however, is that when I am somewhere between 40 and 80 years old, I don't want to hear a doctor tell me that I *need* one of those impressive surgeries in order to live.

It's very sobering to learn that in more than 50 percent of all heart attacks, the first sign of illness is *death.* There are not a lot of great alternatives to that particular health problem. So, in short, I say this: Teach me health. Teach me prevention. Teach me responsibility. And help me apply what I learn.

Although I am making a great effort in this book to educate you about the virtues and value of chiropractic, I do not intend to belittle the value of medicine's vast technological feats. Medicine may have failed at keeping us healthy, but it has many times kept us alive.

Medicine has become a very impressive "repair art" because we are so unhealthy and so often in pain and distress. Repair is the arena in which the medical profession shines the brightest. Medical doctors can repair extreme damage to a person's mangled body, reattach limbs and other body parts, remove life-threatening tumors, transplant organs, reconstruct accident victims, remove bullets, restore electrolyte and fluid balance, fix broken and crushed bones, and repair any number of other horrors that are visited on humankind. These are wonderful and sometimes awe-inspiring examples of corrective procedures.

Once this work is finished by the physician, however, it is the body's life force that takes over and does the actual healing. Your body can, and does, heal itself every day you live. Your magnificent body can knit bones together, heal torn flesh, destroy remaining cancer cells, and restore chemical balance. Even the most gifted medical doctors in the world know that there comes a time when they must stand back and let the body—and a higher power—take over.

Our need for medical doctors is certainly evident. I would never belittle the good things the medical profession does because I believe in giving credit where credit is due—no more and no less. However, I am adamantly opposed to the vast number of misconceptions and the intentionally misleading propaganda being spewed out daily in the media, favoring the medical profession and often denigrating any form of alternative health care.

As you read this book, you might think that I believe we'd be better off without our family doctors and our specialists. That could not be further from the truth. If one day, I pull out into the highway in front of my office, and a huge semi-truck hits me broadside, causing broken bones, profuse bleeding, and loss of consciousness; I want somebody to dial 911 and get me to a trauma center as soon as humanly possible. I want those professionals in the emergency room to do their best to help me—and I believe they will. I am not anti-medicine when medicine is needed. In fact, I applaud many of the medical professional's procedures and abilities. The emergency rooms or the trauma centers of most hospitals have their very best people ready to meet all kinds of emergencies. They are very good at this type of life-saving care.

I still contend, however, that for general health care a medical doctor is not your best choice. After the emergency care for my injuries is complete, and I can be released from the hospital, I will then go directly to a chiropractor to have my body and spine checked for misaligned vertebrae and nerve interference. I want to make sure my body is working at 100 percent of its capabilities because I know the real healing comes from within. If the body still has the innate ability or power to help itself, it will. If the body is in such a weakened, run-down, diseased condition that it is no longer able to repair itself, there is little anyone can do.

That's why we have to work to keep our own internal health system as strong as possible. Our good health is *our own responsibility.* Each of us chooses the path we take on the road to health. There is a road less-traveled to better health, to renewed vitality, and to happier golden years; but we have to make that choice ourselves. Every day you pass road signs pointing you to one road or the other. The direction you take is up to you. After reading this book, you can no longer plead ignorance of what to do about maintaining your own good health. You must realize that you have real choices. You don't have to remain ill, be in constant pain, or die an early and painful death.

This is not to say that this road to good health is an easy one. If you are looking for quick fixes, or short-cuts, you may be disappointed. The road to good health may be very rough at times, but it is not nearly as treacherous or as deadly as the traditional medical route. It is usually difficult to choose the right path in most avenues of our life. We may be able to say "no" to recreational or legal drugs and even pat ourselves on the back for doing so, but it is hard to refuse rocky road ice cream, sausage gravy, delicious pastries, gooey chocolates, morning pots of steaming coffee, an after-dinner drink, or that pack of cigarettes. But it can be done. You hear people say, "these things won't hurt you," and maybe one or two (with the exception of cigarettes) may not do you much harm—but they will do you no good either. It's also not easy to roll out of bed in the morning and take an early walk, to keep a positive attitude, and to remain strong in your convictions, beliefs, and actions. It takes focus and a concentrated effort. What it all boils down to is whether or not we want good health badly enough to strive toward that goal. It's as simple—and as difficult—as that.

Thomas A. Edison, a man who held a vision that surpassed those of almost any other of his era, had this to say about medicine: "The doctor of the future will give no medicine, but will interest his patients in the care of the human frame, in diet, and in the cause and prevention of disease."

Only with the prevention of disease and the maintenance of good health can we finally begin to stop the massive number of bodies floating down the stream. When the members of the medical profession honestly and truly begin to practice the motto of "Do No Harm" and dedicate themselves to seeking the treatment that concentrates solely on "the good of the patient," and when brilliant minds no longer have to consume all of their time "trying to save lives," then, perhaps, we can truly begin to enjoy and appreciate *living* our lives.

# Chapter 2

# What's It All About?

Seems there was this old chiropractor who needed to buy some health insurance. He was told that he would have to have a complete physical exam. The old man was indignant. He'd never been in a medical doctor's office in his life. Since childhood, he had relied on chiropractic care. When he was convinced that he would not be able to get insurance without the medical exam, he reluctantly agreed.

After a few preliminary questions, the examiner asked the chiropractor's age.

"I'm 75 years old," he answered.

"You look about twenty years younger," the examiner said. "Longevity must run in your family." She then asked how old his father was when he died.

"Who said he was dead?" came the reply. "He's 94 years old and fit as a fiddle."

"Wow," the examiner exclaimed. "How old was your grandfather when he died?"

"Who says he's dead?" he again asked. "Grandpop is 114, and he's getting married next Saturday."

"Good heavens," the examiner said, her mouth dropping open. "Why on earth would a 114-year-old man want to get married?"

"Who says he wants to?"

In this chapter I am not going to promise you a certain number of added years. Nor will I claim that chiropractic care, or any alternative or complementary type of health care, will offer you the proverbial Fountain of Youth. What I am saying, however, is that you will live longer, be healthier, and feel better if you are under chiropractic care. Does this interest you?

I will relate the history and methods of chiropractic and allow you to have a closer look at the beginnings of a very simple method of dis-ease prevention. I want to show how chiropractic care has evolved into the largest natural nonmedical healing art in the world.

## WHAT IS CHIROPRACTIC?

The philosophy of chiropractic care is to promote an unobstructed flow of impulses from the brain through the spinal nerves and onward to every cell in the body to help us achieve the balance, harmony, and vitality necessary to enjoy a long, vibrant, healthy, and productive life. Chiropractic is not just for back pain, as has long been the misconception held by many people. It is intended to promote the total health and integration of the body because it focuses on the ability of the body to heal itself from the inside out.

In chiropractic, we refer to an *innate intelligence,* a term that refers to the human body's inherent ability to regulate and care for itself. The remarkable "life force" possessed by the body, as well as its ability to heal its own wounds and mend its broken bones, is the basis for the philosophy of chiropractic. Unfortunately, this belief is also fuel for the critics' never-stopping ridicule of the profession. What is frustrating, however, is that many people never even consider taking the time to really look into the numerous health-care benefits offered by alternative health care because they are ill-informed or convinced that *only* their medical doctor really knows what's good for them.

I often tell people that the goal of chiropractic is to eliminate or reduce the *subluxation.* Most are quick to ask, "What on earth *is* a subluxation?". Some mistakenly believe that removing a subluxation is putting the bone back in place, when it is actually unlocking the malpositioned (subluxated) vertebra from its fixed position, permitting it to move where the body wants it to go. While the chiropractor can make a reasonable determination of the general direction the vertebra has to move, it is *only* the body that knows exactly where the vertebra should go.

In his book *The Confusion About Chiropractors*, Dr. Richard E. DeRoeck summed up the belief behind chiropractic health care very well when he wrote the following:

There is no question that a life force exists in the body. While each of us goes merrily about our business, our bodies quietly manage all the biological functions necessary for us to do so. The heart beats, the lungs breathe, the stomach and intestines digest, the kidneys and liver filter and detoxify, and so on, all without our own conscious control. . . . It is truly amazing.

It is our innate intelligence, or our life force, that guides us throughout our lives. By whatever name it is called—it is as much a part of us as our hearts, our eyes, our minds, or even our souls.

Dr. Herb Schraw, a chiropractic colleague from Toledo, Ohio, spoke at one of my philosophy meetings held last year, and his enthusiasm was extremely infectious.

When the "innate" flow cannot do its job because of a subluxation in the body, it is as though your ability to get well is in prison. The whole concept of chiropractic is to free the imprisoned inside so that man can be in communication with his Creator. Our job is not treating effects—it's adjusting causes, which is the basic difference between medical and chiropractic care.

I think it is very important to emphasize here some of what has convinced me that chiropractic care is necessary to good health. A chiropractor gives an adjustment to a person to provide his or her body with the ability to begin the healing process. This healing process begins at the cellular level. Most of us are aware that every part of our bodies is made up of cells. The chain of cells that make up our bodies are all connected. For example, if the nerve flow to the stomach is being interfered with, the new stomach cells being formed will be inferior in quality. Since the body is constantly repairing itself and constantly making new cells to replace the dead cells, it makes sense that, after a period of time, the stomach as a whole will be inferior since its old cells are being replaced with cells that are not up to standard. You wouldn't replace your old dying sparkplugs with damaged ones, so why would you allow this to happen in your body?

As these inferior cells begin to function improperly, the stomach will weaken, thus becoming susceptible to disease. This disease process causes the symptoms that indicate that there is a problem, which in the case of the stomach are usually gas, indigestion, nausea, pain, burning, diarrhea, and constipation.

When the symptoms get bad enough, the sufferer usually seeks help, perhaps at first from over-the-counter drugs at the local pharmacy. These may bring some relief, but the underlying problem is still there, so the symptoms will return again and again. They will usually get worse until the drug store solution no longer brings relief. The person may then turn to a medical doctor, who, in turn, will prescribe stronger medication to cover the continuing and worsening symptoms. Again, the relief will most likely prove to be a temporary solution. Later, there may be recommended surgery, or if the problem is severe, the consequences could be even more drastic.

If the patient had first sought help for that stomach problem from a chiropractor, the first thing the chiropractor would do is check the spine to see if there was a subluxation interfering with the body's natural ability to function. When this subluxation is found, an adjustment is made to the area causing the particular symptoms, thus correcting the obstruction and allowing the body to begin its own healing. The adjustment releases the nerves that are then able to send the correct messages to the stomach. This starts the process that allows the new cells to be formed the way they were intended, stronger and with more life than the previous cells. As the chiropractic care continues, the interference becomes less and less, and the new cells created become more and more healthy. This allows the stomach to once again start doing its job better, the way the Creator meant it to do it in the first place. This interference will be reduced to whatever level the body is capable of returning to. Unfortunately, this does not always mean a 100-percent reduction because in too many cases, the person has put off chiropractic help for years, causing permanent deterioration and damage. The good news is that the body is an amazing creation that strives continuously to do the best it can because that is the process of life, health, and death. Sometimes even a 50-percent improvement offers a much better quality of life to the sufferer.

If you think about it, our cells are absolutely awesome in their abilities. Each of our cells works tirelessly to keep us going and to keep us as healthy as they can. Some cells in the body secrete enzymes. Some cells help the pancreas make insulin. Some help the hypothalamus control blood pressure, while others keep busy doing a myriad of marvelous things we could never even imagine.

I am still amazed when I stop to consider all the astounding ways the body will work to keep itself healthy, from growing new vessels in the heart to reconnecting severed nerves in the foot. It does all of these things, often in spite of the way it is abused.

We need to do all we can to help this amazing process. This is why people need regular chiropractic visits when they have a health problem. It takes time to correct this life/health/disease/sickness cycle that has been there for much too long—often years. You may think it would take years to correct these problems as well, but often it does not take much time at all to get relief from your symptoms. I cannot stress enough, however, that if you do not fix the cause, your symptoms will return. It may take a while for them to come back, but believe me, they will, simply because they were never gone in the first place. They were just "put on hold."

As chiropractors, we are often berated for having patients return to us for treatment even after their symptoms have disappeared. Regular chiropractic health care is called "prevention," which is a word many people, including those in the medical profession, tend to ignore. It is far better to keep a serious illness from getting the upper hand, than to try to fight a problem that is sometimes beyond the reach of any of the health-care professions.

---

# Did You Know...

... that the most popular form of alternative treatment is chiropractic (used by 13 percent of the American population)? Homepathy is the second choice, utilized by 4 percent of alternative-health-care receivers, followed by acupuncture, naturopathy, and herbal medicine. Almost half of the people who chose alternative care did so because they felt they had not been helped by the accepted health-care system. 70 percent of alternative-health-care patients were pleased with their treatment and considered themselves much improved or cured. Only 1 percent felt their health had not improved.

---

## WHAT DOES IT TAKE TO BECOME A CHIROPRACTOR?

Chiropractors are doctors, though, like dentists, podiatrists, osteopaths, and optometrists, they are not medical doctors. Whether used in connection with philosophy or some other type of study, the term "doctor" indicates a completion of the highest level of a designated area of studies. The advanced professional degree, Doctor of Chiropractic, is conferred upon graduation from a chiropractic college, and is recognized by the U.S. Department of Education.

How little some people know about the years of study we have to complete before we can practice chiropractic never ceases to amaze me. There are some people who have no concept of the intensity of our educational requirements. Some will even wonder why we did not become "real" doctors instead of one of the drugless healers. Some also think becoming a chiropractor is a simple process and takes only a few months of study. This misconception could not be further from the truth.

In order to be granted a license to practice chiropractic, one must (a) be a graduate of an accredited chiropractic college, (b) pass three (a fourth is optional) separate two-day National Board Examinations, and (c) pass a very intense licensing examination administered by the Board of Chiropractic Examiners in the state in which the doctor intends to practice.

In case there are some who also do not realize how much preparation and study are necessary before entering chiropractic college, let's take a look at the requirements needed to obtain the Doctor of Chiropractic Degree. According to the pre-admission guidelines furnished by the Life University School of Chiropractic of Marietta, Georgia, the requirements are as follows:

- A pre-professional background of not less than 60 semester hours or 90 quarter hours, including 6 semesters of writing or communication skills, 3 semester hours of psychology, 15 semester hours of social sciences or humanities, and 6 semester hours of biological sciences, each course with a lab and each passed with a grade of C or better. The biological sciences accepted are animal or human biology (botany and ecology are not accepted as fulfillments of these requirements). Such courses as anatomy, general biology, microbiology, physiology, and zoology are recommended.

- 12 semester hours of chemistry—6 inorganic and 6 organic—each course with a lab, and each passed with a grade of C or better.

- 6 semester hours of physics with a lab and each course passed with a grade of C or better are also required.

- 14 academic quarters of study (4,700 class and clinical hours representing 347 credits) including courses in basic and clinical sciences and other health-related subjects, as well as an internship at either of the college's outpatient clinics. Life Chiropractic College sees an average of 600 to 700 patients *daily* in its outpatient clinics, so there is a lot of hands-on experience during the educational process.

Special emphasis is placed on the relationship between structural and neurological aspects of the body in health and disease. Life University graduates are eligible for licensure as chiropractors in forty-nine states and many foreign countries. The research in which faculty and students engage is designed to provide data about chiropractic phenomena, develop the students' natural talents, and encourage students to accept responsibility for health care leadership.

While it is, of course, possible to obtain a degree and license to practice chiropractic in all fifty states, exact prerequisites for a chiropractic degree may vary slightly from college to college. Because of the difference in state requirements, it would be a good idea to write to the college of your choice asking for full requirements if you are considering a career in chiropractic.

Many people are very surprised to discover the similarities between the education of the chiropractor and the medical doctor. We deal with the same human body, so it stands to reason we would follow most of the same lines of study.

## THE HISTORY OF CHIROPRACTIC

Chiropractic has been practiced for as long as medicine has—actually its use started even before established medicine began. As you will see, there is documentation of chiropractic care being practiced in China many centuries ago. Even when Hippocrates established the practice of medicine, his vision was of a profession more like chiropractic than medicine as we know it today. In this section, we will review the history of chiropractic, from its beginnings in Ancient China, to chiropractic as we know it today.

### Chiropractic Roots in China

One of the oldest recorded spinal adjustments comes from ancient China. A series of drawings on turtle shells revealed that more than 4,000 years ago, spinal care was practiced in China. An historian cites an ancient document from China believed to have been written about 2700 B.C., in which manipulation of the spine is clearly described.

Most historians are familiar with China's extensive knowledge and implementation of alternative health care. Chinese medicine has much to teach us about many types of health care—some of which may seem very strange to those of us in the Western world. It teaches that the relationship between the mind and the body is very important to our good health and well-being. Much of Chinese medical therapy is based on herbal treatments, acupuncture, and massage-related treatments, and has been administered for thousands of years. Its positive effects have been well-studied and documented.

China is well-known as a forerunner in the field of massage. Massage is considered a complement to the standard medical treatment in China. Chinese masseurs are not doctors, but their work is considered a specialty. It is not simply a technique for loosening the muscles or relaxing stiff joints, it is designed to release the flow of *chi*, or the life force. These masseurs use their hands to help put the body back in balance. They search for the root of whatever problems beset the patient.

When journalist Bill Moyers was touring Chinese hospitals, doing research for his book *Healing and the Mind*, he asked one of the doctors why a woman who was suffering pain from fibrocystic breast disease was having her *back* massaged.

"Because her breast problem is caused by obstructed chi in her liver," was the answer given by the doctor. He continued to explain by telling Moyers that following the line of the *meridian*, he was working on her inner organs in order to recoordinate her chi and blood, thereby treating her disease. "That is why she needs to be massaged," he said, "not locally, but in areas far away [from the affected area]."

When Moyers asked how the doctor knew the chi was stuck in the liver, the doctor explained that there were symptoms and physical signs that could be located through the sore points in her back and where the meridian was weak. In short, massaging her back affected the liver, and the liver affected the breast. It was also explained to Moyers that in Chinese medicine, the meridian is believed to connect the interior and the exterior portions of the body, thus our inner diseases can be treated through the exterior of the body. Once the chi of the meridian is opened up, the disease is cured.

There is no doubt of the effectiveness of this form of treatment because manipulative treatment has been practiced in China for centuries. The practitioners have a saying that is very familiar to those of us in chiropractic: "Where there is an obstruction, there is pain. Once the obstruction is removed, the pain disappears." Sounds simple doesn't it? Actually, it is very simple, and very effective.

Chinese hospitals even have massage units in addition to surgery or orthopedic units. Can you imagine our hospitals having a wing for chiropractic health care? I can, I do . . . and we will.

## Chiropractic in Ancient Greece and Rome

An early Greek papyrus, dating back to 1500 B.C., gives instructions for maneuvering the lower extremities to treat lower back conditions. There is even a rare early Greek work known as the Edwin Smith Surgical Papyrus, which was studied by Greek and Roman physicians some 1700 years before Christ, that describes a back sprain and instructions for manipulating it.

As mentioned in Chapter 1, Hippocrates, the man who has been called The Father of Medicine, was a sincere advocate of spinal care. There is recorded proof that Hippocrates is only one of many physicians and practitioners who, for centuries, valued the healing power of spinal adjustments. Further studies of history show us that some form of chiropractic (by various names and labels) has been practiced in nearly every culture known to humankind, with its roots extending back to the beginnings of recorded history.

Hippocrates taught his students how to reduce a posterior spinal curvature caused by a fall as follows: "The physician, or some person who is strong and not uninstructed, should apply the palm of one hand to the hump, and then, having laid the other hand upon the former, he should make pressure, attending whether this force should be applied directly downward, or toward the head, or toward the hips." Hippocrates also designed the first table for making spinal adjustments, fitted with various pulleys and clamps that enabled the physician to make effective adjustments with minimum risk to the patient.

There have always been people who recognized that an intimate relationship exists between the spine and good health. Evidence suggests that spinal care goes back to a time long before medical care existed, and has been one of the more favored systems during our civilized existence.

Another great name in healing is Claudius Galen (A.D. 129–199), the most famous physician of the early Roman Empire. Galen was among the first to recognize the importance of the nervous system. He also discovered seven of the twelve important cranial nerves, as well as the cervical, lumbar, and dorsal (thoracic) regions of the spine. He is credited with giving the first recorded chiropractic-style spinal adjustment to one of his patients, Eudemus.

Eudemus was a Roman scholar whose fingers were paralyzed, and Galen diagnosed the problem as arising from impinged (pushed together) nerves in his neck. After his neck was adjusted, Eudemus was elated to discover the numbness had disappeared. The doctor was just as pleased as his patient and became a strong advocate of spinal adjustments, believing that "leaving the affected parts alone, you will reach the spine, from which you will treat the disease." He also taught his patients and students to "look to the nervous system as the key to maximum health." Now, I ask you, does that sound familiar?

## Early Manipulative Arts in Europe

Although many European physicians did employ the manipulative arts during various periods of time in history, the practice was not as widely used there as it was in Asia. Unfortunately, after the fall of the Roman Empire in A.D. 476, spinal manipulative art was almost forgotten or the practice was lessened by most European physicians during the period known as the Dark Ages. Twenty centuries of accumulated human knowledge disappeared into oblivion as hundreds of libraries were destroyed and thousands of scientific documents were burned by invaders. Fear and superstition replaced scientific inquiry and understanding in the Dark Ages. The development of manipulation was almost lost because the popping sound was thought to come from the demons who were causing the disease in the first place. Only those known as folk healers kept spinal manipulative arts alive as they traveled about the country practicing (often in secret) a form of chiropractic procedure known as *stamping* or *trampling*. The preferred method of treatment for the medical doctors of that era was the use of chemical solutions, pills, and potions, often making the treatment far worse than the problem.

The trampling procedure was similar to the method used for centuries by Japanese women who practiced backwalking to provide relief from stress and sickness. This was another form of manipulation that gave comfort to those on the receiving end of the backwalker's talented feet. Some countries, it was said, even used large bears to do the walking, a procedure I think might be a little unnerving, depending upon the attitude and personality of the bear. Backwalking is still practiced by the Maori peoples of New Zealand.

In ancient Hawaii, a form of manipulation called *lomi-lomi* was used to heal the sick. It was first discovered by Europeans in the seventeenth century when their ships encountered the Polynesians.

By the late Middle Ages, Europeans were enjoying a resurgence of spinal manipulation. The procedure became very popular during the Renaissance, when it was known as *bonesetting*. Those who were called *bonesetters* practiced throughout the towns and villages of Europe and Asia. Using knowledge handed down from one generation to the other, these early practitioners were regarded as gifted healers who could treat a number of illnesses by manipulating bones back into place. Spinal manipulation was often successful when other methods failed. By the eighteenth century, bonesetting was one of the most recognized healing arts throughout Europe. One of the most famous practitioners in this country was a man named Steven Sweet, who resided in Long Island, New York and came from a long line of bonesetters.

The January 5, 1865 issue of the *British Medical Journal* contained an article written by renowned British surgeon, Sir James Paget entitled "Cases that Bonesetters Cure," which extolled the benefits of bonesetting. In 1925, the British medical journal *Lancet* carried an editorial about England's most famous bonesetter, Sir Herbert Barker, giving the chiropractic profession still another complimentary pat on the back: "The medical history of the future will have to record that our profession has greatly neglected this important subject (manipulation) . . . the fact must be faced that the bonesetters have been curing multitudes of cases by movement (manipulation)."

## Spinal Manipulation in the New World

While Asia and Europe are rich with the history of spinal manipulation, the procedure certainly was not unheard of in the New World. It was practiced in one form or another by the Winnebago, the Sioux, the Creeks, the Incas, the Toltecs, the Tarascans, the Zoltecs, the Aztecs, and the Mayans before European settlers arrived.

## Nineteenth Century "Discoveries"

Though long understood and treated by ancient medical practitioners, another "discovery" was made by the medical profession in the early nineteenth century. It was called *spinal irritation*. The concept was that problems arising in the spine or spinal cord caused many different diseases—fever, coughs, stomach disorders, lung problems, vomiting, colic, asthma, diabetes, and menstrual disorders. The diagnostic symptom was tenderness upon pressure over a vertebra. This diagnostic procedure that was once used by ancient practitioners is still used today by chiropractic clinics all over the world.

And how did the medical community handle this discovery? By using adjustments to treat these problems? Well, not quite. Preferred medical spinal treatments, unfortunately, involved none of the things a bonesetter of the day would have done. Medical spinal treatments often defied logic. One such treatment involved the application of hot irons to the skin over the tender spinal areas. Let it suffice to say, not many people responded well to this harsh treatment, and it is doubtful that many patients returned for treatment. This was a very good example of the treatment being far worse than the problem. Other doctors used yet another strange and unusual treatment for the spine. Instead of applying a hot iron to the patient's back, they applied leeches to suck the blood out of that particular area. Again, not a picture you'd want on the brochures you put in your waiting room.

Overall, the medical profession has skirted around the methods of chiropractic, some of which were so successful, some doctors adapted these methods for their own practice—and as a result were ostracized by their own profession. Those doctors who were brave enough to seek chiropractic care for themselves or their families were in grave danger of being discovered and severely disciplined by the medical community.

## Early Chiropractic Care in America

It was a hot summer afternoon in Davenport, Iowa in the year 1895 when Daniel David (D.D.) Palmer, who was referred to as a nonmedical healer or a magnetic healer (one that heals by laying on of hands), listened to a man tell about an accident he had suffered eighteen years earlier. Harvey Lillard, a deaf janitor, told Palmer that he felt "something give" in his back just before losing his hearing.

Palmer asked Lillard to lay down on a bench so he could examine his spine. During Palmer's examination, he found a misaligned vertebra. He placed his hands over Lillard's spine and gave three short, quick pushes. By the third push, he heard a faint "click" from his patient's back.

In his 1006-page text *The Science, Art and Philosophy of Chiropractic*, published in 1910, Palmer further described his encounter with Lillard:

> Harvey Lillard, a janitor in the Ryan Block, where I had my office, had been so deaf for seventeen years that he could not hear the racket of a wagon on the street or the ticking of a watch. I made inquiry as to the cause of his deafness and was informed that when he was exerting himself in a cramped, stooped position, he felt something give way in his back and immediately became deaf. An examination showed a vertebra racked from its normal position. I reasoned that if that vertebra was replaced, the man's hearing should be restored. With this object in view, a half-hour's talk persuaded Mr. Lillard to allow me to replace it. I racked it into position by using the spinous process as a lever and soon the man could hear as before.

The account went on to relate that after three adjustments in three days, Lillard jumped up from the cot and cried out, "Doc! Doc! I hear!" To Lillard it was nothing short of a miracle that for the first time in seventeen years he could hear the sound of the horse-drawn trolleys on the street four stories below. Even though Palmer was aware that he had indeed helped a "miracle" to occur, he probably didn't realize at that particular moment the revolutionary effect this simple act would eventually have on the field of health care.

Convinced at first, that he had found a cure only for deafness, Palmer began to practice his "hand treatment," as he called it then, on other patients. When it was discovered that a patient who had suffered from heart trouble was also relieved, he was even more amazed and excited. Word spread of this new drugless healing method, and people came from all over the area. They reported being cured of stomach trouble, skin conditions, sciatica, headaches, asthma, and any number of ailments. D. D. Palmer became known as the discoverer of a powerful new drugless way of healing. Palmer became more and more aware of his place in history. He had this to say about his fame: "I am not the first person to replace subluxated vertebrae, for this art has been practiced thousands of years. I do claim, however . . . to create a science which is destined to revolutionize the theory and practice of healing art."

One of Palmer's early patients was a minister named Samuel H. Weed who had studied the Greek language. Weed is credited for the naming of "chiropractic." The Greek word for hand is *cheiros*, and *pracktos* is Greek for "done by," thus the combination of the two words formed the word "chiropractic." Up until this time, this remarkably effective form of health care with ancient beginnings had been called by many different names.

While Palmer lacked formal education and many were not impressed with his views on holistic health, he never stopped believing in or practicing his healing art. At the same time, he was a strong-willed and overly suspicious individual, who did not really want to share his discovery with others. He wanted to keep it in the family. However, his son, Dr. Bartlett Joshua (B.J.) Palmer, ultimately convinced him to establish the Palmer Infirmary and Chiropractic Institute in Davenport, Iowa in 1897. The school, which was the largest of its kind, featured a three-month course and attracted a diversity of students including several women, medical doctors, surgeons, and osteopaths. Among the students was Dr. Alfred F. Walton, who taught at the Medical College of the University of Pennsylvania. Dr. Walton, a graduate of Harvard University Medical School, became one of the school's most impressive alumni and supporters of the positive effects of this *new* form of health care. He lectured and wrote extensively in support of chiropractic care and helped to give it respectability in the eyes of many of his peers and the general public.

B. J. Palmer, who is also considered a very important figure in the history of chiropractic, was only 14 years old at the founding of the new healing art. He did not have a happy childhood, and his father, while a great visionary, was less than desirable as a parent and a business partner. The father/son combination was a classic example of a love/hate relationship. Even though the two strong-willed men worked together, theirs was a volatile partnership that was never completely resolved. As a result, the younger Palmer was left with many problems, both personal and financial, after the death of his father in 1913. Nevertheless, he believed strongly in the method of chiropractic, and, in spite of an extremely difficult life, he never wavered from his goals.

During his lifetime, B. J. Palmer patented over 100 inventions and owned the first radio and television stations west of the Mississippi River, in addition to his chiropractic practice and the running of the school. He was quite convinced that this thing called a "subluxation" was the basis for the healing art, and he took the time and money to research it, even though he was constantly being labeled as unscientific and foolish. He set out to prove the naysayers wrong—and he did. Palmer also believed that his ultimate purpose in life was to leave behind a great legacy—not an estate nor hordes of money—but the legacy of having touched a large number of lives in a positive way. He died in 1961, leaving both of these legacies behind him.

Dr. B. J. Palmer was the first to teach that the term dis-ease does not mean "disease" in the sense that we know it, but rather, it refers to a lack of harmony (or ease) within the human organism. He defined dis-ease as "that condition which allows illness (or disease) to exist: It is dis-order and mis-alignment." Palmer went on to point out that dis-eased bodies all have one thing in common—they are not working correctly and are, therefore, malfunctioning in their area of weakness. He believed that disease attacked areas of weakness, not strength.

## Chiropractic Care Today

Chiropractic is now the largest drugless form of health care in the Western world. It often gets results where other methods fail. Its practitioners are the best trained in their field and provide an impressive and successful health-care service for numerous ailments.

We see amazing results in our offices every day as chiropractors. Nothing better proves that a patient's physical condition has improved than when the patient actually feels better. Nothing offers greater case results than a patient who has been given up on by the medical profession, but after turning to chiropractic is now living a healthy, pain-free life. Chiropractic care and other alternative methods of care and prevention are continually gaining ground and will ultimately become the primary health-care leaders of the future.

Why do I believe this to be true? Because there is a growing number of patients who are becoming disenchanted with the medical profession as it exists today. They are searching frantically for a method that will work for them, and many are finding it in chiropractic care.

In 1990, Americans made 425 million visits to the so-called "unconventional" alternative health-care providers (including chiropractic), while only 388 million made visits to primary care physicians and medical doctors. It would seem that people are turning away from the "conventional" caregivers in great numbers.

Why is this happening? People are realizing that organized medicine is not really working the way we've been led to believe it is. I believe that in the near future the insurance companies will make sick people go to a chiropractor for a second opinion before they will allow (pay for) surgeries or permit (pay for) unnecessary and costly medicine to be prescribed. This would be one of the most positive things that could happen in the health-care business. People would be healthier, have fewer surgeries, take less medicine, and save money to boot.

Chiropractic is also gaining acceptance in the medical field. We still have a long way to go, but I am pleased to report that more and more medical doctors are learning that chiropractic care is very important in the total healing of a patient. Many physicians no longer hesitate to refer their patients to a chiropractor or to seek chiropractic treatment themselves.

From time to time chiropractor Dr. Herb Schraw visits a medical college in Toledo, Ohio to listen to lectures about medical care and new methods of treatment. He was amazed by some of the comments he heard there recently. "I sat in on lectures for a total of eight hours," Dr. Schraw said. "There were about sixty medical doctors who were discussing basic [new] things that we, as chiropractors, have known for years. Out of the ten speakers they had, orthopedic- and neurosurgeons, can you guess what every single one of them talked about?"

"Subluxations?" I asked.

"Subluxations is right," he said. "Every one of them mentioned 'subluxation,' not once, but several times. I can even quote one of the neurosurgeons who said 'subluxation is progressive and can cause neurological and cord compression, and certainly neurological compression is potentially life-threatening.' Imagine that. Hasn't anybody been listening to us all these years? Are they just now learning what some ancients knew centuries ago?"

Although chiropractic is widely accepted today by those who are educated about its numerous benefits, we still must continue to try and get this important message across to everyone.

In a 1994 two-hour NBC-TV special, *Cured! Secrets of Alternative Healing* (in which chiropractic care was neglected, I'm sorry to say), surveys were done of people who use various alternative methods to "regain control of their own health and not be passive to a doctor." Among the subjects discussed were herbal treatments, acupuncture, mind-body healing, and homeopathy. To balance the report, so-called "experts" were presented who spoke both in favor and against the alternative methods.

It was clearly evident that some of the medical doctors were completely closed-minded about any form of treatment not compatible with their own views and personal opinions, while others showed an extremely open attitude about the various options. One doctor in particular was against all alternative methods. "Wasn't possible," he said about the effectiveness of some methods. He was positive that there was no such thing as chi— "Doesn't exist." He sneered at the word meridian. "No such thing," he said with absolute certainty. None of the alternatives worked. He was sure of it. He was absolutely positive that his opinions were, indeed, fact, and he was not open for further discussion of any alternative method.

In watching the program, I was reminded of the man who was asked directions to a nearby town.

"Oh, there is no road," he told the inquirer. "You can't get there from here."

A little boy standing nearby spoke up and said that yes, indeed, there was a road. It was not known by a lot of people, but he had traveled on it, and he knew it existed.

"Oh, no," the man scoffed in the boy's direction. "There is *no* road. *I've* never seen it. *I've* never traveled on it. It doesn't exist."

It didn't exist *to his knowledge.* For some people, just because they've never traveled a road—never needed to journey to a particular place—maintain emphatically that it does not exist.

## The Old and Improved

Greatly improved and refined since 1895, the art of chiropractic adjustment has relieved numerous varied problems, including musculoskeletal (muscle/bone) and visceral (organs) conditions. It has also kept many patients healthy at a reasonable cost, without the use of drugs and/or surgery. In addition, it has been successful in helping our bodies control such disorders as hypertension, rheumatism, bronchial asthma, arthritis, allergies, nervous tension, chronic fatigue, heart trouble, and a host of other ailments, some of which do not respond at all well to medical intervention.

When there is a problem, and you correct it, it is easy to claim victory; but when you prevent a problem from occurring, it is quite difficult to prove that you have prevented it. For example, if you decided to leave for work thirty seconds earlier one morning, and a truck came barreling through an intersection that, had you left at your regular time, you would have been right in the middle of, and probably would have been killed; you do not know for a fact that your life was saved because you left thirty seconds earlier. Your fortune would probably be attributed to a host of other factors as well. However, if you had been there at the time the truck came through, your survivors would probably lament that if you had left home thirty seconds earlier, you would have avoided the accident. Likewise, if you take care of yourself—watching your diet, exercising, and getting chiropractic adjustments—and you manage to avoid cancer and other serious ailments for most of your long life; rather than attribute your good health to preventative care, people will probably just call you lucky. But if you do get ill, your loved ones will wish that you had done something to prevent it. Prevention should be our goal in health care. After all, it's a whole lot smarter (and easier) to take care of yourself so you don't get sick than it is to take care of yourself once you've become sick.

Even if you have not endured a lot of pain and illness yourself, you probably know people who have. It's a terrible thing to watch another person suffer. We fear pain and suffering, yet we do very little to prevent it. It is only when we are in pain that we seek relief. How much simpler—and better for us—it would be to prevent illness from happening in the first place. We have to give our bodies every chance at wellness that is known—and we know that chiropractic works. We know that regular exercise works. We know that a well-planned, healthy diet works. We must start making better choices. We must take better care of ourselves, and then we will enjoy better health later—guaranteed. It's a simple life principle.

## DOES CHIROPRACTIC GUARANTEE A STATE OF POSITIVE WELLNESS?

To a large degree, yes, I do believe chiropractic offers an assurance of wellness. However, you must also realize that heredity, diet, and exercise play important roles in your health as well. But with regular chiropractic care, your body will work and function the way it was designed to. There is no other form of health care that even begins to address your overall health and prevention of illness the way chiropractic does.

The goal of chiropractic care, again, is to lay the foundation for positive wellness and general well-being by keeping the nervous system free from obstruction by spinal misalignments. Chiropractic is about prevention of illness and getting rid of pain. It's about good health. It's about an alternative to drugs and surgery. It is a welcome addition to many other forms of treatment. Whether you are enjoying good health and want to maintain it, or are concerned about a problem that does not respond to conventional treatment, you need to be informed. You need to know there is an alternative.

Never make decisions based on assumptions. Always check

out the facts about any new treatment you are considering. Talk to people who have had long-term experiences with chiropractic health care. Learning about chiropractic care may be one of the most important things you can do for yourself in your lifetime—which, I hope, will be as free of pain and disease as possible. It's your life. It's your health. It's your choice. Not many things are more important than your good health or your choices about how to achieve it.

It is entirely up to *you!*

# Chapter 3

# What to Expect When You Go to the Chiropractor

*Once upon another time, there were three handsome young bulls—a very large one, a medium-sized one, and a small one—all walking down a quiet country lane. As they walked, they discussed the real meaning of life.*

*Suddenly, over to his right, the big bull noticed a lush green pasture. Within the fences were several very attractive cows. He was very impressed and announced to his companions that he had found the true meaning of life. Without another word, he jumped gracefully over the fence.*

*The other two walked on.*

*A little later they approached yet another pasture—even greener and with even more beautiful cows. The middle-sized bull nodded in that direction and told the little bull that he, too, had found the place he wanted to be. He jumped the fence and was welcomed into the herd.*

*The little bull continued to trudge on down the country lane for the remainder of the morning, all afternoon, and on and on into the dark of the night. No one really knows just how far this little fellow walked, but everybody knows that a little bull can go a very long way.*

It was Marie Curie who said that nothing in life is to be feared, it is only to be understood, which I think is considerably closer to the truth than former President Franklin D. Roosevelt's oft-quoted words, "The only thing we have to fear is fear itself."

As a chiropractor, it is often surprising for me to discover
that people are almost always apprehensive about coming to
me for the first time. Some have confessed later that they were
actually frightened. Very few people come to a chiropractor's
office the first time with even a smidgen of understanding as
to what will happen, and all of them watch me like a hawk
all through the initial visit. There are times when I feel almost
as though I'm on stage the way some new patients watch my
every move and try to read my expressions to determine if I'm
an OK guy who actually knows what I'm doing. They seem to
be afraid I'll say or do something *weird*. They want assurance
that they are in the right place, that it is OK for them to be
there, and that everything is going to be all right. In other
words, they're afraid . . . of me. I am not to be feared. I am
only there to help. Some are heeding the strange and unusual
things they've heard about this type of health care. A little bull
does go a very long way, and often becomes quite exaggerat-
ed. Is this what makes us afraid? Or is it simply that we fear
what we do not understand?

That little bull just keeps on walkin'. That's what all these
stories are—pure bull. Many more people know that now, but
because of old habits and fears, they are still going to watch
and ask questions—something I welcome wholeheartedly.

I recall one patient who told me that he came to me for help
in spite of the fact that his doctor had told him *not* to go to
a chiropractor. I wanted to find out why the doctor told him
this, so I called the doctor. I asked him if he'd ever been to a
chiropractor's office. He said he had not. I asked him then if
he had ever watched a treatment, or even spoken to a chiropractor. He had done neither. I invited him to my office. He
didn't come.

For a time I continued this practice of calling a patient's medical doctor each time the patient said that he or she was advised not to see a chiropractor. Each time the result was the
same. No return phone calls. Nothing. None of them would
agree to discuss chiropractic care or to come to my office to
observe firsthand exactly what I did. Evidently, they saw no
reason to find out anything more about this drugless form of
health care that helps millions of people every year.

What did this tell me? For the most part, it told me that

these medical doctors I spoke with thought they already knew it all, didn't care, or were convinced that what medical school had taught them about chiropractic was true. All that the medical doctors were doing when they advised their patients not to utilize chiropractic care, was parroting what they had been taught in school by another medical doctor, who was taught the same thing by another medical doctor, who was also taught the same thing, and so on, and so on. The bull just goes on and on. Millions of people (including medical doctors) have been misinformed and continue to suffer because of uninformed people feeding a little bull to others about chiropractic care.

If we would take the time to think rationally about chiropractic care, then we would lose many of our fears. Think of this, for example. In 1895—when chiropractic was founded—if those first 1,000 or 1,500 people who utilized this care had gotten hurt, been conned in any way, or not been helped, what do you think would have happened? Would chiropractic have continued to grow and flourish, in spite of the massive and unrelenting attacks against it by the medical profession and drug companies? No way!

Today, chiropractic is the largest natural healing profession in the world because it works. It helps people. Those first patients way back in 1895 got better. They got positive results! So, by word of mouth, from those who knew that chiropractic care provided the health benefits that it claimed to provide, this health-care profession was established. Millions have been helped with their pain and incapacity, and people who had suffered needlessly began to get blessed relief. What more could a patient want or ask of his or her health-care professional?

You would think that since patients don't have to worry about getting stuck with a needle, having harmful medicine prescribed, or being scheduled for dangerous surgery, they would approach chiropractic care with an open mind and with hope, especially since the vast majority have already been to their medical doctors for their problems prior to seeing a chiropractor. They should approach it with the hope of stepping onto the threshold of a new health-care system. Every chiropractic office in the country should be filled—not with sick people—but with people striving to maintain better health.

When new patients come to my office, I try to set their

minds at ease from the beginning. I give them extensive questionnaires to answer—not because I'm nosy—but because the more I know about them, the more I am able to help them achieve the healthy state they deserve. Most of my patients have questions for me, as well, and I enjoy this exchange. Often it takes a few visits before they feel comfortable, but I am confident that most of them will soon be at ease with me and my treatment. The more they know about me and my methods of chiropractic, the better they will be able to help me to help them.

This chapter will answer some the many questions I am asked by my new patients.

### Why won't some people go to a chiropractor?

Too many people are uninformed, frightened, or have not been in enough pain to seek relief, and as a result do not go to a chiropractor. Those who have been told by their medical doctors not to go to a chiropractor may never seek the help they could find there because they believe their family doctor knows best. Some do not come because their insurance companies are so short-sighted and uninformed that they do not cover chiropractic care. Again, we are allowing money people to control our health care.

However, the most common reason people fail to go to a chiropractic physician lies at the chiropractors' feet. We do not tell the story often enough to let more people know that there is an alternative to pill-popping and surgery.

### Why do people go to a chiropractor?

Unfortunately, many people go to a chiropractor as a last resort, having spent years going through pain, aggravation, and expense before finally throwing up their hands in surrender and trying a chiropractor. Pain (usually back pain) is the number one reason people go to a chiropractor especially for that first visit. It is rare for a patient to learn of the numerous advantages of having a healthy spine and top-performing immune system, and then come into the chiropractor's office asking to begin a program in order that he or she may enjoy a lifetime of disease prevention.

Patients usually show up at my office because some friend or relative told them how much they had been helped—when nothing else worked—and how much better they feel now that they are going to a chiropractor regularly. Some come because they've heard chiropractors can get rid of migraines or arthritis, or because they knew someone who got relief from severe menstrual cramps. They may have suffered a fall or a car accident. They may have had a problem with a stiff or painful neck, a whiplash, a sports injury, digestive problems, or even fatigue, but they almost always come because they are hurting and want relief. A friend or relative could not stand to see them suffer anymore and insisted they give chiropractic a try. Nothing spreads faster than word of pain relief.

Fortunately, more and more knowledgeable, enlightened, and open-minded medical doctors refer their patients to a chiropractor when their treatment has failed. This is good news for the patient because a doctor who will look at all aspects of the person's health is a doctor who cares about the individual. The bad news is that there are still many medical doctors out there who are too closed-minded to consider chiropractic as an alternative.

### Does a chiropractor treat all those disorders you talked about?

A chiropractor treats only the spine. The goal of the chiropractor is to activate your inner doctor by helping you achieve a healthy spine, which will activate your body's own natural healing ability. The body can and does heal itself if you remove the interference!

People often think that they are going to the chiropractor for treatment of headaches, vision problems, leg pain, or whatever their symptoms may be. That is not completely accurate. The chiropractor corrects spinal stress (vertebral subluxations), one of the most deadly and most destructive blockages of life and energy from which we can suffer. It is when this problem is corrected that the other symptoms go away.

### What is a vertebral subluxation?

A subluxation is the misalignment of one or more vertebrae causing nerve interference.

## What causes vertebral subluxations?

There are lots of answers to this question. Some vertebral sub-luxations can be traced back to the process of being born, others back to childhood accidents, and others to more recent trauma. These are referred to as *macro-stress*. The second kind of vertebral subluxation cause, *micro-stress* is caused by repeated movements that gradually wear down your body parts. Things such as poor posture or the repeated movement of a certain part of the body—as in certain occupational activities—can cause vertebral subluxations.

Many people do not realize that certain emotional stresses can inflict more damage upon the spinal column than can a serious automobile accident. This is why we advise the general public—and certainly our patients—to let the chiropractor help you fight the slow onset of chronic diseases.

## How do subluxations cause interference in the flow of nerve transmissions?

The misalignment causes the opening between the vertebrae—through which the nerves travel—to be narrowed, causing the interference of transmission of messages between the brain and the rest of the body to occur within those spaces. Scientific research has shown that the weight of a dime on the nerve root can cause up to 60-percent less flow of nerve transmission.

When your body's communication system is out of order and the messages cannot get through, sometimes you are fortunate enough to have your body tell you—through pain or other symptoms—that something is amiss. Other times you may have the problem and be totally unaware of it until it becomes extremely serious—even past the point of correction.

Let me give you an example of what I mean. Steven was a 10-year-old boy. He was the proud owner of a new bike that he received for his birthday. He loved to ride fast, do wheelies in front of his girlfriend Lauren's house, and show all his friends how well he could ride.

Steven didn't pay too much attention to the sidewalk in front of him, however, and he hit a big rock in his path. He and his bike went airborne and landed at the bottom of the hill. The bike had a few broken spokes, and Steven was covered with cuts and bruises, not to mention the wounds to his ego. He even cried a little. But he was young and strong, and he didn't cry long. He bounced back quickly, even though he was terribly sore and stiff the following day. A few days passed, and he appeared to be as good as new. The bike wreck was forgotten, except when he wanted to boast to his friends about how high he flew into the air.

Steven and his parents were unaware that the accident caused a lower neck subluxation. No one thought of taking a 10-year-old boy to a chiropractor. He didn't even go to a medical doctor, so why should he go to a chiropractor? He showed no signs of head injury or broken bones, so there was no need for any kind of treatment. You know boys. They have their falls. No problem.

Steven's body then had to handle this subluxation the best way it could, which meant adaptation. And luckily, the body is pretty good at this, even on its own. The body compensated for the subluxation for as long as it could, and on the surface, all was well. Steven was a healthy boy, and both he and his bike were both soon back in good working order.

When Steven was 15, he would sometimes complain of some stiffness in his neck for no apparent reason. "Oh well," his parents thought. "He's an active boy. Things like this happen."

By the time he was in college, Steven was having headaches quite often and was still bothered by a stiff neck. But he learned to live with it. The idea of connecting any of these symptoms to that long ago bike wreck never crossed his mind.

When Steven was 35, he found that he was suffering more and more from unexplained numbness in his arm, which concerned him quite a bit. A friend recommended that Steven see his chiropractor, and Steven decided it wouldn't hurt to try—it might even help.

It did help. The chiropractor found the subluxation that had taken place twenty-five years earlier, and he went to work trying to correct the subluxation as much as possible. It couldn't be totally corrected with one or two visits, but with regular adjustments over time, it continued to heal. It will probably never be 100-percent back to normal because of the length of time the cause (injury) was allowed to remain. But with proper care, Steven will at least *feel* 100-percent better and will have little or no symptoms. His lower neck will be an area of weakness in his body now (due to twenty-five years of degeneration), and he should take care of it with periodic chiropractic checkups.

How much better it would have been to have had this checked out by a chiropractor when Steven was 10 years old, and he could have avoided many of the problems he had encountered during the years that followed.

Misalignment can also occur without causing nerve damage. Scoliosis (curvature of the spine) is an example. You may have scoliosis and be subluxation-free in the areas of curvature, but you will most likely have subluxations in some other part of the spinal column.

### Does everybody have subluxations?

Yes, nearly everyone is affected by subluxations at some time in their lives—and most do nothing about it—ever. Even more distressing is that most don't even know about them—what they are or the damage they can do.

One analogy likens subluxations to termites. Not a great thought to picture little creatures eating away at your insides, is it? Subluxations are burrowed into your spine, much the way those pesky little insects are burrowed into your house. By the time the termites eat through your floor joints, and you fall through your bathroom floor, a tremendous amount of damage has already been done to your house. Likewise, by the time you feel the pain in your back, there may have been a long-standing subluxation silently devouring your spine, and, unfortunately, a complete recovery may not be possible.

I have never examined anyone over the age of ten, who wasn't already under chiropractic care, who did not have one or more subluxations. This is why I constantly stress the importance of a periodic spinal exam in order to locate and correct vertebral subluxations.

### Can I tell if my back has a subluxation in it?

You cannot always tell if there is a subluxation in your back. I will use a dental cavity as an example. A problem may be forming inside your tooth, long before you are aware of it. When you finally go in for a checkup, your dentist looks in your mouth and asks if you've had any pain or adverse reactions to hot or cold foods. You say you haven't. Then he probably wants to take an x-ray. When he shows you the x-ray, he points out that he has discovered a cavity and may explain how he will drill in your tooth to fix it. He doesn't come back to you and say, "Well, Mrs. Jones, there's a cavity in your tooth—here it is on the x-ray—but since it's not hurting, come back and see me when it begins to ache. Of course, at that point, I may have to pull it, instead of just filling it."

You wouldn't have a lot of confidence in a dentist who said that, would you? It is not smart to put off fixing a problem until you are in pain. You know it can only get worse, so it makes no sense to wait for a bad toothache before you to try to get it fixed. Again, I must bring up the old ounce of prevention slogan . . . it's worth "a pound of cure" or a ton of pain. This is why I encourage my patients (and others) to get periodic examinations and adjustments of the spine. It's your health and prevention of dis-ease we're talking about.

### Are subluxations the only causes of nerve transmission interference?

Though vertebral subluxations are the most common forms of interference in the nervous system, there are many other causes as well. Most drugs work by altering the chemistry of the nervous system, which, of course, affects the function of the nerves. Aspirin, for example, and other analgesics work by interfering with the flow of the nerve pain messages. Other things that cause damaged nerves are burns, freezing (frostbite), and severe cuts. Poor posture can cause nerve pressure, like when our legs "go to sleep," lack of blood supply to the nerves is most likely causing this uncomfortable situation.

One of the most dramatic kinds of deterioration due to nerve transmission interference is seen when someone suffers a stroke. A blood vessel in the brain is blocked or bursts, and this deprives a particular area of blood and oxygen, causing both the nerves and the muscles they serve to deteriorate, often beyond the body's ability to repair itself. Broken bones; arthritis; tumors; or neurological diseases, such as muscular dystrophy, multiple sclerosis, polio, and cerebral palsy can also adversely affect nerves.

*How long does a spinal adjustment take?*

After the chiropractor is familiar with the patient's spine, it usually takes only a few minutes to make a spinal adjustment. It also depends on the adjusting technique the chiropractor is using. Some techniques take very little time to perform—just seconds—some take longer. The key is to remove the nerve interference, no matter how long it takes.

Some complain when they have to pay the chiropractor for a ten or fifteen minute visit. Once a medical doctor has completed his or her examination, he or she decides on the course of treatment—a shot, a prescription, or suggested bed rest. How long does it take to give a shot, scribble a prescription, or give a pat on the shoulder? Would you want a shot to take thirty minutes, so you could feel you got your money's worth? I don't think so. A chiropractor treats patients in exactly the same manner. As soon as I complete my examination and decide what the patient needs, the proper adjustment only takes a few seconds. Remember, whether you are at your medical doctor or a chiropractor, it's not how long it takes, but whether the treatment is done correctly that will make the difference.

*Does a chiropractic adjustment hurt?*

A chiropractic adjustment does not hurt. You will be able to feel the adjustment, and often you'll hear the click, but it is a drugless, painless method of health care. What could be more natural than that? You must realize, however, that often chiropractors see people who are already in a great deal of pain, and sometimes, simply touching these people causes more pain. The adjustment itself, however, does not hurt.

*How dangerous is a spinal adjustment?*

A spinal adjustment is not dangerous at all. Chiropractic is among the safest and most gentle of the healing arts. After almost 100 years of attacks from the medical profession, the charges of chiropractic being dangerous have been proven to be unfounded. Compare malpractice insurance rates of chiropractors with those of other health-care professionals, and you will find that malpractice insurance rates for chiropractors are only a small fraction of those in the medical field. This is because the malpractice insurance companies wind up having to pay out so much more money for those in the medical field than for those in chiropractic.

Respected medical authority, Robert Mendelsohn, M.D., once said, "When the AMA hollered about 'unproven remedies,' 'extravagant claims,' and 'unscientific methods,' I thought they were referring not to chiropractors, but to it's own M.D. members."

It would seem that with all the pain, suffering, and deaths caused by the medical profession (see Chapters 1 and 12), the American Medical Association might just want to soft-pedal on the subject of dangerous treatments.

### What is that "click" sound made during a spinal adjustment?

Not all adjustments or all techniques used by chiropractors produce the click, or popping noise, you may hear. Most patients say the noise is similar to the sound produced when one "cracks one's knuckles."

The sound can probably best be explained by the results of a test performed by a British research team a few years ago. The team took x-ray movies of a person "cracking" his knuckles, and found that gas (80-percent carbon dioxide) rushes in to fill a partial vacuum created when the joint surfaces are slightly separated. This slight separation of joint surfaces also occurs during a spinal adjustment. It is believed that this displacement of joint fluid causes a gaseous release and causes the "cracking" sound in a spinal adjustment as well. If you crack your knuckles twice in a row, you won't hear a second pop because the gas will have dissipated.

### Can I crack my own neck?

When a person cracks his or her own neck or back, it is not the same thing as when a chiropractor makes an adjustment. The act may relieve tension for a little while, which may give the person the false impression that it helped him or her. However, if you feel that your neck or back needs "popping," it is usually because a part of your spine is fixated or jammed, causing another part to move too much and pop a lot—sometimes by itself. The jammed or fixated part should be properly adjusted *by a chiropractor* so the rest of the spinal column will stop being so movable and noisy.

When a person starts trying to manipulate themselves, they usually have to do it more and more often. It almost becomes a nervous habit. That's because you are unable to adjust yourself properly. A chiropractic adjustment is not a do-it-yourself procedure anymore than is open-heart surgery. A chiropractor cannot even adjust him- or herself properly. I go to a chiropractor on a regular basis and would not even consider doing my own adjustments. Anyone who feels he or she needs to crack his or her neck or back needs chiropractic care. That's their bodies' innate way of telling them that something is wrong and needs help.

Your grandmother probably used to tell you that cracking your knuckles could cause arthritis or make them bigger. While there has been no research done to support that notion, it's probably best not to argue with Grandma.

### Are there any side effects to chiropractic care?

There *are* side effects to chiropractic care. In fact, there are many side effects to spinal adjustment. If you come in for treatment of pain in your lower back, or perhaps for treatment of a shoulder that has been giving you some problems, you will be given an adjustment to help that particular area to heal itself. What you may not realize is that during the time you are getting the adjustment, your sinus problem is clearing up (coincidence?), you have fewer headaches (more coincidence?), you no longer are as fatigued or have trouble sleeping. You may think you simply feel better, and you do. The fact that your back is better and/or your shoulder no longer aches, is credited to your chiropractor, but you don't think of the fact that he or she could have something to do with the disappearance of your other symptoms. Those are the "side effects" of chiropractic care, and there certainly may be many others—all *positive.*

### Can chiropractic care be utilized instead of surgery?

Many times a patient comes into my office because they can't stand the thought of surgery. Even if I were not a chiropractor, I could certainly understand this fear. If surgery does have to be performed, and there are cases in which it is necessary, it should be the absolute last thing considered. There are many, many times that patients have come to me because they were scheduled for surgery, but they wanted to "try chiropractic" first. They were later elated to discover that surgery was no longer necessary.

Back surgery, especially, can be prevented by a chiropractor. In the majority of cases, painful and dangerous back surgery becomes unnecessary once a patient is under chiropractic care. Many doctors honestly tell their patients that, even after back surgery, the problem may remain or could come back. The fact is, it could be even worse after surgery. With chiropractic care, we believe that in most cases, the treatment will help the patient to avoid the surgery completely. I would think this one single benefit would be enough of a reason for most patients to check into chiropractic care before submitting to back surgery of any type.

### What if I've already had back surgery . . . is it too late for chiropractic?

It is not too late to consider chiropractic, even if you have had surgery. It may, in fact, be very important that you seek chiropractic care for any further problems you may encounter. Many patients who have had spinal surgery often find that their painful back problems return months or years later. For this condition, doctors can now bill a patient's insurance company for a condition they have created—*FBSS*, or *Failed Back Surgery Syndrome*.

Fortunately, people who have had back surgery can receive chiropractic care without worry, and may be saved from further surgeries. Most people who have had back surgery are not anxious to repeat the experience. Each case is an individual and it is a good idea to make your chiropractor aware of as many facts of your history as you can.

### How many times do I have to go to the chiropractor?

There is no "magic number" of times you must go to the chiropractor. How many times do you go to have your teeth checked? How often do you have your eyes examined? How many times will you have to go to a medical doctor? How many pills will you have to take? How many surgeries will you have to endure? How many years have you been in pain?

Chiropractic is not a "patchwork" treatment, although many approach it as if it is. It should be a lifelong commitment to your own good health. Some people may only go once in their lifetimes. Once is better than never, I suppose, but that is not health care. Fortunately, for some people, their spinal problems may be nothing more than a slight misalignment, rather than long-standing nerve stress, and one visit may seem to take care of the problem. When you find a chiropractor with whose abilities and reputation you feel comfortable, you can trust him or her to tell you exactly what your overall health-care needs are, and how to achieve the best quality of health care possible.

Most people think they will have to go to a medical doctor for the rest of their lives—and even more often as they get older. We have to wonder why so many people are surprised to discover that chiropractic is not a one-time healing procedure. If you stop going to a chiropractor, spinal stress will start, or continue, to build up as it did before you utilized the care. It will have no way of being reduced, and, therefore, your health will be at a much greater risk.

Chiropractic care is a safety valve, releasing pressure from your system. If that pressure stays high, with stress unrelieved, your good health will suffer. If the pressure is relieved, your system will revert to the way it was created to work in the first place. It's really quite simple if you think of it in these terms.

A chiropractor's office should seem neither strange nor mysterious. This type of image contributes to one of the greatest health misconceptions we have today. There are so many people who are sick, tired, and suffering, living on painkillers or other drugs, and perhaps facing life-threatening surgery who could be helped with chiropractic care, yet do not go because of lack of knowledge or understanding, or because of fear.

### Is chiropractic care addictive?

Chiropractic care *is* addictive. It is addictive in a very positive way. You'll really love doing something for yourself that is good for you. You will love how much better you feel, and you will want to continue feeling good. You will know that your general health is improved. That is the kind of addiction we should all have.

Actually, chiropractic is not physically or even psychologically addictive, but once you discover for yourself how much better you can feel and how much your general health can improve, and you begin to educate yourself about the benefits of chiropractic care, you will want to return again and again, as needed. Furthermore, you will want to keep yourself on a regular preventative maintenance schedule, the same way you go to your dentist, your medical doctor, or your optometrist regularly. Doesn't it make more sense to want to *stay* well than to try to *get* well?

"Is chiropractic addictive?" If only it were . . . a little. There would certainly be a lot fewer sick people if chiropractic visits were among everyone's ongoing health-care habits instead of something we do when our backs are "killing us."

### Do I have to get x-rays?

Unlike Superman, we cannot see into, or through, a patient. The x-ray tube, invented in 1895 (the same year chiropractic care began) by William Roentgen, is a trusted and necessary tool for a chiropractor. Chiropractors have used x-rays as an aid to diagnosis since the early years of its existence.

Chiropractors use x-rays to analyze the spine's alignment and posture and to detect spinal curvature caused by scoliosis, kyphosis, or lordosis. It is also used to detect indications of spinal degeneration or osteoarthritis, as well as broken, fused, oddly shaped, or malformed bones. It can also show bone spurs and other problems, which will help us to perform an effective spinal adjustment. It helps show us what we can do, as well as some techniques not to use, on individual patients. It continues to be the most popular tool for both a chiropractic and a medical doctor's spinal analysis. While I certainly do not recommend repetitious x-rays, I do find them to be extremely useful, especially at the beginning of treatment. There have also been some cases in which, with the use of an x-ray, I have discovered broken bones in patients, a condition that should be treated medically.

Recently, a registered nurse came in for an appointment because she had been involved in an automobile accident about two-and-a-half weeks prior to her visit. She had been treated at a local hospital emergency room where she was employed, x-rayed, and released. Her pain was still severe, more than two weeks later. During our initial consultation, I realized something wasn't right. With years of experience, you notice degrees of pain, and hers appeared to be excessive, especially considering the time her body had had to heal. Imagine my surprise and her shock, when I found, after taking x-rays, that she had a broken neck. Needless to say, this was a medical emergency. She was admitted to the hospital immediately, put into a brace, and surgery was performed the next day. X-rays are necessary (and in many cases, life-saving) and allow us to help the patient by actually "looking inside."

X-rays are simply a diagnostic tool. They are not a see-all, tell-all device, but they do help the chiropractor analyze the spine for areas of probable subluxation. We take hard tissue x-rays, not soft tissue x-rays. We look for spinal misalignment, which causes nerve interference. In order to have a more complete spinal analysis, other analytical procedures and tools—such as MRI (Magnetic Resonance Imaging) and CAT (Computer Assisted Tomograhy) scans—may be used. We use whatever necessary methods to find out what is causing discomfort, pain, or disease in our patients.

*How often do chiropractors refer patients to medical doctors?*

We refer patients to medical doctors as often as it is necessary. Chiropractors believe in doing what's best for the patient. We know there are times when surgery is necessary, and so are certain drugs. We also know that patients want and deserve the best and most effective way of dealing with their illnesses, and sometimes it is necessary to refer the patient to a medical practitioner. The ideal situation for a patient is to have a great medical doctor and a great chiropractor, *both* concerned about keeping the patient in optimal health. Your medical doctor and your chiropractor should be on the same side, for the good of your health!

*I've heard that chiropractors are only after your money. Is this true?*

A good chiropractor's first priority is the patient's good health. I'm aware that there are those who say we are only after the money. This is also said about those in the medical profession. Every profession has people whose sole purpose in life is to make a buck one way or another. But for every one like that, there are thousands of others who have a genuine interest in the "patient-first" concept. I believe that, basically, people who choose health-care professions want very much to help people.

To answer the question directly, yes, I do think there are some chiropractors out there who are working only for the money. They are the ones I call "money people," who hook you up to unnecessary machines, take too many x-rays, or have you come in only until your insurance runs out. Fortunately, these people make up a small minority of chiropractic doctors, but in my opinion, one is too many! You should never feel uncomfortable with any treatment given you by any type of health-care practitioner. If you do feel as though you are being taken advantage of, get a second opinion or switch providers.

The main reason some patients feel they are being ripped-off by chiropractors is because they don't understand chiropractic care. Chiropractors need to do a better job of educating our patients about what to expect and why. You see, we can only help you when we see you! We don't send you home with an armload of drugs to get you through the pain, we work "hands-on" to improve your health. Medical doctors give you drugs for ten days or so before you return to be rechecked. Actually, the pill you're taking four times a day is a treatment. We don't ask you to come into our offices four times daily, but sometimes we do need to see you as often as three times a week, especially at the onset of a serious problem. It amazes me that people will undergo a dangerous surgical procedure costing $20,000 with no guarantee, yet will balk at chiropractic care three times a week for four weeks, which will cost them about $400.

### Will my medical insurance cover chiropractic care?

There was a time, not long ago when insurance companies considered chiropractic a nonentity and refused to pay any coverage for chiropractic care. Fortunately, they have kept abreast of the studies done by workers' compensation groups that prove that with chiropractic care, people return to work sooner, avoid lengthy hospital stays and costly surgeries, and, overall, spend less time and money on their illnesses. Many insurance companies now provide for a preventative once-a-month chiropractic visit, and even more if there has been an injury. Restorative chiropractic care is often covered by Medicare and Medicaid in many states, and most private insurance companies now include chiropractic in their policies. There are still unenlightened companies that fail to recognize the savings chiropractic care could afford them and their clients, and as a result, will not pay for chiropractic treatment. I suggest you shop around for an insurance company that recognizes the importance of alternative medicine.

### Why don't chiropractors work in hospitals?

Chiropractors do work in hospitals in some areas. There are more places now than ever where chiropractors have hospital privileges. It would be wonderful to see everyone who was admitted to a hospital checked for spinal nerve stress and subluxations also. If anyone needs a chiropractor, it is those people who are experiencing life-threatening diseases.

There has been some indication that the medical profession is considering giving chiropractors even wider hospital privileges. Unfortunately, there would most likely be many compromises to be made on the part of the chiropractor. What the hospitals are discussing is not adding the knowledge and talent of the chiropractor to their teams, but rather, implementing the medicalization of the chiropractor's patient. This would involve chiropractors referring their patients to medical doctors in order to have medical tests and treatments performed, rather than medical doctors referring their patients to chiropractors to have spinal adjustments performed—which would make a lot more sense.

### How soon should I start my children on chiropractic care?

I believe you should offer your children chiropractic care as soon as possible. If your newborn has gone through an especially difficult or traumatic birth, it would be advisable to get him or her to a chiropractor right away. This is especially true if the child cries more often than your first child did, is far more fretful than your brother's newborn, or is generally an all-around cranky baby. It could be that this child is trying to tell you something, because his or her little body is trying to tell him or her something.

If the thought of having your baby's back adjusted bothers you, please understand that the adjustment for an infant is far different than it would be for an older child or an adult. Their tiny bodies are treated gently and with the utmost care. One trip to the chiropractor will convince even the most particular of parents. Most techniques used on babies are so gentle, it almost looks like nothing is being done. You'll hear no popping sounds when a baby is being adjusted. The issue of child care is discussed in much detail in Chapter 9.

### Can you be too old for chiropractic care?

You cannot be too old to benefit from chiropractic care. Chapter 10 is devoted to discussing the care of older chiropractic patients. Many elder patients have suffered through the "drug maze" and fought their way out of it with the help of a good chiropractor. What we must do is better educate our older family members about chiropractic care, and make sure they know how it can improve the quality of their golden years. People, especially older people suffering from bone disease or osteoporosis, need special spinal care if they are exceedingly brittle, but a trained chiropractor is very much aware of these problems, and works with the patient accordingly.

Although chiropractic is called a "healing profession" or a "healing art," it still makes no claim to heal the disease. I think it has been made pretty clear that, basically, a chiropractor adjusts your spine in order to help your body to be able to heal itself. Removing the interference to the nervous system allows the energies of life to flow through the body providing nourishment, flexibility, strength, and balance—enabling your inner doctor to bring about the healing your body needs. It is as simple, and as miraculous, as that!

# Chapter 4

# The Back Bone's Connected to the Hip Bone

*One fine day, it occurred to the members of The Body that they were doing all the work, and Belly was getting all the good food without much effort. So they held a meeting and, after a long discussion, decided to go on strike 'til Belly consented to take its proper share of the work. Then, for a day or two, Hands refused to pick up the food, which meant that Mouth no longer had to receive it, and, of course, Teeth and Throat no longer had to chew or swallow.*

*However, after a while the members began to find that they were no longer feeling very active. Hands could hardly move, Mouth was parched and dry, and Legs were unable to support The Body for any length of time. They discovered that even Belly, in its own quiet, dull way, was doing necessary work for the body, and in order to survive, all must work together, or The Body would go to pieces.*

—Aesop Fable

One of the most prevalent ailments in our society is back pain. You can hardly go through a day without someone mentioning (too often at length) how bad his or her back hurts. When your back hurts, you can hardly think of anything else. It is only natural that you will share this misery with others, whether they want to hear about it or not. When someone says they "hurt all over" when they have a backache, they probably mean it, since the back affects almost every other part of the body.

When someone says they have a bad back, lower back pain, a slipped disc, or a pinched nerve, their problem is usually not that simple. There are so many kinds of back problems, that it would be difficult to list them all. There are also as many different opinions as to what the treatment of each one should be. What we do know, however, is that these back problems are all connected. Like the old spiritual song says—the hip bone's connected to the back bone, the back bone's connected to . . . and so on. What affects one, affects another. In fact, everything in the body is connected to the back in one way or another.

Most people are prime candidates for low back pain. It is one of the most common complaints. You can hardly get through the day without seeing someone reach back with both hands, push down on the lowest part of his or her back, make an ugly face, and wish aloud for some relief from the obvious discomfort that they are experiencing. At the same time you hear the complaints, you usually hear their opinions of the cause of the problem as well.

"Must be gettin' old."

"I need to get more exercise."

"Oh, man, I played softball yesterday . . ."

"I've been sitting too long at my desk."

"I've been driving too long."

"I'm so stressed out with all the things going on in my life."

"The kids are driving me crazy."

"The boss is giving me a headache."

"Guess I'll have to give up being a couch potato."

Do any of these reasons sound familiar? Sure they do. All of them are common "causes" or reasons for back pain. Sometimes, one or all of the reasons can be the culprit. The reason could also be an injury of some type that was never properly diagnosed and treated.

Back pain, we all know, is not fun, and, perhaps, neither is this chapter. But let's hang in there together and see if we can learn something about these bones of ours, that, once connected, can "get up and walk around," as the song goes.

## COMMON CAUSES OF BACK PAIN

We suffer lower back pain because the lower back, or lumbar spine, bears most of the body's weight, making it vulnerable to injury and pain. The underlying cause of back pain is a misalignment (subluxation) of the bony framework of the body.

As is the case in an office or a factory, there are always those who have to do more than their share of the work. This is the case with the lower back as well. Our Creator knew that much pressure, stress, and strain would be exerted on that area, so the lumbar spine was made bigger and stronger to compensate. The structure of the lower back is not disturbed by simple everyday activities, such as making the bed, washing your hair, or bending over. However, while it's not very easy to injure your lower back, it does happen. Daily, in my office, a patient with lower back pain will tell me they don't know what happened to cause it.

"I must have slept funny because it hurt when I got out of bed."

"The pain just started in my lower back for no reason."

Their backs did not start hurting because of the way they slept or for no reason. In all likelihood, most of their lower back pain was caused by some type of injury or trauma in their past, perhaps even years ago. Something happened to their back that was never fixed, and is now showing up to cause all kinds of trouble.

There are several things that can be done to prevent some back problems. There are exercises you can do to strengthen the spinal muscles. Weak, flabby, underexercised muscles contribute greatly to low-back problems—but then, so do overexercised muscles. Muscles subjected to the same stresses and strains every day will lead to back troubles, if there is a subluxation present. When you are tired or emotionally drained, you are more prone to injury. Stress takes its toll by keeping your muscles shortened, tense, and tightened.

What I'm saying is that in today's busy world with its often hurried lifestyle, low-back pain is very common. The pain may indicate a problem within the structural elements of the back itself, or it may be sounding an alarm for another part of the body. If you suffer from low-back pain, a subluxated vertebra is usually the culprit.

I must warn you that you should not try to diagnose your own back problems. It's human nature to try to do that, but it's not a good idea. Mild low-back pain may be ignored and/or explained away for years, but you know that is not smart at all. This is an area that needs your utmost attention and care. Do you honestly think that your back is going to get *better* with age? Sometimes, a few weeks or months may pass, and it may feel a little better, but you can count on the return of the pain, each time with more intensity. Common sense will tell you that. Common sense should also tell you that you should not have to put up with low back pain when it can be avoided with the help of your chiropractor.

Your chiropractor can pinpoint the cause of your problem or problems with a thorough examination, which may include the use of x-rays and other tests. Evaluation of the cause of lower back pain precedes the necessary spinal adjustments to relieve the problem. It can also help the chiropractor to discover some problems that may require medical attention.

## Pinched Nerves

The preferred technical terms for a pinched nerve are *nerve irritation, nerve impingement, foramina compression, nerve-meningeal tension, spinal stress,* or *neurothlipsis.* In other words, the term "pinched nerve" is actually interchangeable with the term "subluxation." Regardless, people will still say that they have a *pinched nerve* because that's what it feels like. In many cases, people with pinched nerves may not be in much pain at all, especially in early subluxations. Because of the body's ability to adapt to the misalignment, they can be totally unaware of the problem. Pain is only one symptom of a vertebral subluxation. The reason for the lack of pain in many cases is because only sensory nerves carry pain messages. If these sensory nerves are not badly damaged, then no pain will be felt. While damage to the nerves and other tissues may be occurring, there will be no pain to warn the unwary victim. People with painful pinched nerves are the fortunate ones because they are made aware of a problem in their spines and can take the necessary steps to get themselves checked out by a chiropractor.

The saga of the pinched nerve is not all that complicated. If all is well, the nerve fibers in your body begin their journey from the brain where they originate, heading for their final destination. They usually travel in bundles bound tightly together (then called nerves) and once packed up, they go merrily on their way.

First, they go through a large hole in the bottom of the skull, and then travel through the spinal column as part of the spinal cord. When they reach their exit, which is a hole located between the vertebrae, called the intervertebral foramina, they head for their final destination.

Upon leaving the spinal column, the nerves change modes of transportation. They split up from the large bundles and begin to branch out into smaller and smaller bundles until they complete their journey into every little small town and hamlet (nook and cranny) in the body.

The journey is successful when there is no pinched nerve. But if the vertebral misalignment is even slight, it may cause the nerves to be irritated, compressed, or stretched. The openings, or foramina, that the nerves travel through may slightly alter in size and put pressure on the contents. To put it simply, the exit is clogged by an obstacle in its path, and the nerves are unable to complete the journey they began. Nerves aren't the only things in the affected area. There are blood vessels, lymphatics, meninges, fat tissue, discs, ligaments, joints, muscles, fasciae, tendons, and other connective tissue, all of which may be affected. The nerves are "compressed," along with other tissues in the foramina, and the communication train is derailed. It cannot complete the journey, and therefore the body is subjected to problems caused by this breakdown in the system.

## Slipped Discs

The term *slipped disc* is really a catch-all phrase for many back problems. The truth is, there is really no such thing, since a disc cannot actually slip. It is knitted into the vertebrae from both above and below, preventing slippage of any kind. It is the vertebrae that sometimes slip out of position and put pressure upon the disc, contributing to its damage, that causes the problem. Regardless of what we call it, a "slipped disc" is probably one of the most painful things that can happen to your back.

At least 85 percent of those diagnosed with a slipped disc

respond readily to chiropractic adjustments. Granted, sometimes there are some protruding discs that are misaligned directly against the nerves that may require medical treatment. But fortunately, this is not a common occurrence. Even in these extreme occurrences, chiropractic care is extremely helpful even after surgery.

## Ruptured Discs

*Ruptured discs* can occur when either the disc between two vertebrae breaks off and irritates nearby tissues, or a disc's soft center oozes into places where it should not be. Fortunately, this condition is not a common occurrence. Spinal discs are, however, constantly subject to gravity and torque from body movements and are susceptible to wear and tear from day to day activities. Some people blame disc problems on "old age," but many are surprised to discover that signs of degeneration can show in people as young as their teens, and I have seen x-rays of people in their nineties that showed little or no signs of disc degeneration.

Spinal misalignments caused by accidents, improper lifting, or sprains may cause the disc to bulge, herniate, or impinge upon a delicate spinal nerve. Even the slightest misalignment can produce nerve interference that may surface in a variety of symptoms and effects. A good example would be an impinged nerve in the lower thoracic (midback) region, which can cause localized pain or weakness in an organ that this particular nerve services, such as the colon. Constipation, colitis, or other digestive problems may result right away or even after a longer period of time. Any impairment of the proper flow of energy through a nerve is usually followed by a malfunction in the organ it serves. Chiropractors can provide relief to herniated disc sufferers by adjusting the subluxated vertebrae, allowing the body to begin the healing process.

## Scoliosis

Although everybody wants to have good posture and a straight back, the average spine is not perfectly straight. It usually curves slightly to the right or to the left. There is sometimes some twisting (rotation) of one or more vertebrae. When the spine curves excessively, it is called *scoliosis*, which is from the Greek word for "crooked."

In the majority of the cases of scoliosis, the cause is unknown. In 10 to 15 percent of the cases, the specific cause is tumor, infection, a neuromuscular disease such as cerebral palsy or muscular dystrophy, a deformity at birth, or disc problems. It was once thought that poor posture was one of the causes of scoliosis, but that is no longer believed to be the case. Some contend that scoliosis is hereditary, while other studies point to possible emotional factors. As you can see, the most consistent thing about scoliosis is that there is little agreement on the exact cause. The good news is that 90 percent of minor curves do not get any worse.

The treatment of scoliosis causes even further disagreement. Some use the bracing method for treatment, while others opt for electrical stimulation. Still others (usually surgeons) argue that neither has any value to the patient, and would probably recommend surgery. Often rods are inserted into the back as a treatment for scoliosis, which often causes constant pain and irreparable damage to the spine.

While scoliosis is not a life-threatening disease (many people live out their lives without knowing that they have it), it is often painful, and severe cases can cause impaired respiratory or heart problems. Since most cases of scoliosis are not considered serious, many believe that the overtreatment of this mysterious ailment is almost as bad, if not worse than, the actual problem. I do not think that it is a good idea to subject any patient with scoliosis to surgical procedures, or even bracing, without first exploring all of the less radical alternatives such as chiropractic treatment.

Dr. Robert Mendelsohn, author of *How to Raise a Healthy Child in Spite of Your Doctor* writes:

Epidemiological studies on scoliosis are so scanty that we know next to nothing. There are no prospective controlled studies regarding the effects of orthotic treatment on the natural history of idiopathic scoliosis. . . . Is anything actually prevented or is progression merely delayed until a later period of life? The answers simply are not known.

The most recent research on scoliosis shows that the cause, or at least an important contributing factor, is a disturbance or a defect in the area of the nervous system that controls posture, body balance, and positioning. Correction of spinal nerve stress would certainly improve the problem, since the nervous system must remain free of structural damage in order for the body to function in a healthy manner.

What it all boils down to is that our body is perfectly designed. All the bones, nerves, and muscles are connected together in such a way that it works. It really works well if all systems are in the proper order and alignment, which is the sole purpose of regular chiropractic care.

## Arthritis

Arthritis is a painful condition that can affect any joint, but is particularly painful in the back. It is another condition that many people simply write off as a problem of old age, and they live with it the best they can. Sadly, I've found that too many medical doctors will tell the patient that their back pain is caused by arthritis and give him or her a prescription for pain medication to get that patient to quit bothering them and accept that pain as inevitable. As soon as patients hear the word "arthritis," all too often they accept that they must live in pain. Not me. I don't accept any kind of pain as the way things are.

Granted, arthritis is no small matter, especially to those who suffer from it, but it is not brought about by old age. It is caused by injuries or mechanical stress (overuse or improper use) of the joints. As we get older, there is a greater chance we will suffer from these things, but it is not really an "old-age disease," as we are taught.

Chiropractors have many patients who suffer from arthritis. Not only does chiropractic care correct misalignments caused by the minor injuries (which can cause arthritis and osteoarthritis), but preventative chiropractic measures greatly reduce the chance of developing these diseases in the first place.

I would implore you to never give up and never accept less than a pain-free life. Life was meant to be wonderful. The first step in achieving that is believing it!

## Muscle Pain

There are other muscle afflictions similar to arthritis, such as chronic muscle spasms, fibrositis, fibromyalgia, muscular rheumatism, myofascial syndrome, and myositis. None of these are pleasant and they are easily misdiagnosed and mistreated.

Did you ever notice what animals do upon waking from a nap? They stretch their backs, their legs, and their necks before taking a single step. Animals realize that their muscles are a little stiff after prolonged rest and immediately try to stretch their muscles out to increase the blood circulation in those muscles.

How do you feel when you first get out of bed in the morning or when you get up from your easy chair after an evening of reading or watching television? Are your muscles tight? Are there aches and pains in the back of your neck? Does your lower back feel heavy? Are you unusually stiff? These and several other symptoms, such as morning fatigue and tender points on your body, let you know you are suffering from any one of the previously mentioned disorders.

What's in a name? Not much. A rose by any other name would smell just as sweet, and pain feels the same no matter what you call it. You can call your chronic muscle spasm "honey," but it won't make it any better—and people may question your sanity.

Six million people, mostly women, between the ages of 20 and 50 are diagnosed every year with one of these conditions affecting the muscles (usually one condition—different name), and it is believed they represent only a very small fraction of those who are actually suffering from these ailments.

Those who suffer from muscle disorders describe it as constant pain between the shoulder blades. Sometimes the neck, shoulder, hip, or lower back aches without ceasing. There are other times when the arm or leg is numb, tingles, or hurts. It may be caused, in part, by emotional stress, arthritis, poor posture, locked spinal joints, or poor eating habits. (Yes, that can cause it too.) Again, the patient may complain that "everything hurts," and all of these aches and pains are almost always accompanied by chronic spasms and constricted connective tissues. Unlike the family cat, there is no way you can "stretch" it out on your own, but it might help.

Our bodies are 60-percent muscle and bone. The 650 or more

muscles that are connected to our bones are called skeletal or striated muscles. They do our work for us, but they tire easily. Sometimes we don't let them rest—or we let them rest too much—and the result is pain and tightness in our muscles.

Wrapped around the outside and lining the inside of muscles and nerves is a strong sheet of connective tissue called muscle fascia. Fasciae, which look like cellophane, carry the many nerves, blood vessels, and lymph vessels that nourish the muscles. Chronic muscle problems result when the fasciae are damaged and the blood, nerve, and lymph supply to the muscles are interrupted.

Doesn't that make sense? No? Well, let's try this. Nerves make the muscles move. They also supply muscles with growth nutrients. Cut a muscle's nerve, and it becomes paralyzed and withers away. Just as when a person is being fed through a feeding tube. Cut the tube, and soon they will wither away and die.

Even though standard medicine is stumped by the actual causes of muscle spasm, fibrositis, and other causes of pain in the muscles, medical treatment includes injections of pain-numbing agents such as Novocain (procaine hydrochloride) and Xylocaine (lidocaine), cooling sprays, muscle relaxants, and cortisone. Some of these medications make the pain disappear for awhile, while others do not help some people at all. Sometimes the patient feels even worse and is referred to a physical therapist to be treated with heat and massage—some of which can offer temporary relief.

Chiropractic care involves removing the subluxations, which can alter concentrates of enzymes and other chemicals necessary for skeletal muscle health.

## NECK PAIN

Sometimes neck pain can be explained—and treated—very easily. Other times, it is quite serious and complex. Most of us have had a pain in the neck at one time or another. No, I'm not talking about the woman down the block who drops in unannounced and never knows when to go home or a brother-in-law who always just needs ten bucks to tide him over.

A pain in the neck is—well, a pain in the neck.

It is a serious place to have a pain. The neck is such a vital

---

# *Did You Know...*

... that in 1971, the state of Oregon's workers' compensation department gave proof that chiropractic is not to be underestimated? Patients with comparable back ailments were used in a study conducted by Rolland A. Martin, M.D. In his study, 82 percent of chiropractic patients returned to work in one week, but only 42 percent of medical patients returned to work in one week. Suffering and expense were drastically cut with chiropractic care as well.

---

part of our body, and if its nerve functions are interrupted, even for a few seconds, we lose consciousness. A little longer, and we die. There is no situation more serious than that. The creators of the old western justice system knew that a rope around the neck was a quick and sure way to punish that horse thief or the stagecoach robber. The neck is home to blood vessels, nerves, the thyroid and parathyroid glands, the larynx, the esophagus, the trachea, the brain stem, the spinal cord, the spinal column, and the meninges. Is this serious, or what? In addition to housing and protecting these very important occupants, it holds up your head and permits it to turn, tilt, and bend up and down. The Latin word for neck is "cervix" which means a constricted area. Seven neck vertebrae numbered cervical 1 (C-1) to cervical 7 (C-7), support the head.

If you carried a ten-pound weight around all day, you know you would be extremely tired. Imagine how much more fatigued you would be if you tried to carry it with your arm extended way out from your body. This is how a fatigued neck can feel if your head is not properly balanced. Your neck will suffer from fatigue as well as stress. So, it might be well to give your chiropractor credit for helping you "keep your head on straight."

## Whiplash

Whiplash is a very real problem. It can happen easily and is extremely difficult to correct. Even a minor fall, a misstep, or a slight bump of the automobile you are in by another automobile can cause a great deal of trouble and may be the cause of even greater problems in the future, some of which can be very serious. What's even more tricky about whiplash is that you may feel perfectly fine at first, yet weeks or sometimes months later, you realize that you are far from being all right.

Although whiplash most often affects the neck, there is certainly more to it than neck pain. Whiplash happens when tiny displacements of the bones in the neck and back occur, brought on by the "whipping" action of the head and neck. Pain from these injuries can occur throughout the entire body, from head pain to sciatica, which can reach all the way to your toes.

I saw firsthand how whiplash happens one day while I was stopped at a traffic light. I happened to look over in the lane next to me and saw a friend of mine, Dr. John Kelly. I was waiting for him to look in my direction so I could wave at him when a car hit him from behind. It was really nothing more than a bump, with no damage done to either car, but I'll never forget the incredible whipping motion made by his head and neck as the other car hit his. His head was first thrust backward, then forward again in a matter of seconds. I never realized how lethal this injury could be until I saw it with my own eyes. Dr. Kelly's neck was sore and painful for weeks. I could only imagine how much worse his neck would have been had the other car been traveling at a higher rate of speed. So the next time you dismiss somebody who complains of whiplash—just hope you never have to find out yourself that it is, indeed, a very real problem.

No area of the body is spared by whiplash. Ligaments, muscles, nerves, and blood vessels (all known as soft tissue) are stretched and injured. These are very slow to heal, often leaving scar tissue as they do that will cause you problems for the rest of your life. Neck pains, headaches, sinusitis, insomnia, allergies, shoulder pain, arm pain, facial pain, or even chest pain are only a few of the many problems connected with whiplash. Furthermore, the danger of degenerative arthritis is a very common long-term effect of this seemingly minor injury.

Anyone who has had a whiplash injury, no matter how small you might think it is, should immediately go to a chiropractor to have his or her spine checked for a subluxation. If you don't do this, the potential for future problems are great. In short, there is no such thing as "just a whiplash."

## Other Neck Pain

There may be several different causes for one's neck pain, among them irritation, inflammation, injury, and infection. Another cause for neck pain can be disc degeneration somewhere in your back. Your medical doctor may write off the cause of this as aging, since the contributing spinal imbalance, spinal nerve stress, and excessive physical or emotional trauma tend to accompany advancing years; but it can be found in the young as well.

Arthritis is another culprit in neck pain. Normally, the neck has a backward curve, but the spinal curve may reduce, becoming what is called a "military neck." An unhealthy neck can often curve in the wrong direction. In time, arthritis can set in, causing changes in the vertebrae such as lipping or spurring (bony outgrowths of different shapes); disc thinning; or degeneration of the muscles, ligaments, and other structures. This was once believed to be a permanent disability, but the good news is that recent studies have shown that chiropractic care can actually reverse some of the effects of osteoarthritis.

Damaged or irritated nerves from a fall, a whiplash, spinal nerve stress, emotional stress, or poor work habits can also cause neck problems. Problems in the neck can cause you to suffer from dizziness; ringing in your ears; headaches; nasal problems; facial pain; throat and tongue problems; or pain in the shoulder, arm, wrist, hand, or fingers, among other symptoms.

The medical approach to neck pain involves the use of painkillers, tranquilizers, muscle relaxants, cortisone, neck pillows and collars, traction, and/or surgery. I know firsthand that an adjustment by your chiropractor is the answer to most neck problems. Medical doctors and physical therapists are not trained to locate and correct spinal nerve stress. As a result, your problems could continue for years after an accident or trauma, and medication to deaden the pain may become a way of life for you. Without proper chiropractic care, the injury may continue to cause damage during this time. By the time the source of the problem is recognized, it may be too late to repair even half the damage done.

Sometimes your medical doctor will refer you to a physical therapist. They are very helpful in the rehabilitation of many muscular conditions, which is where their focus lies. However, if a misaligned vertebra is causing your symptoms, you must have chiropractic care in order to fix the cause. Physical therapy exercises can help you strengthen the spinal muscles, but if the spine is misaligned you would be strengthening the muscles to hold the bone in the wrong (misaligned) position. The reason many people have health problems directly related to accidents that happened years ago is because the underlying cause (subluxation) was not fixed in the first place. The symptoms were treated instead of the problem.

## SHOULDER PAIN

Only the lower back causes us more problems than do our shoulders. And—surprise!—some problems in the back can affect the shoulders. The shoulders can be affected by neuritis; bursitis; neuralgia; rheumatism; or sprained, strained, or sore muscles. Our shoulders are often subjected to much abuse because they are in constant use. An injury to the shoulder often affects your arms and hands as well because—guess what— they are all connected! The shoulders are closely related to the spinal nerves that originate in the neck and, therefore, affect the neck and all of its complex problems as well. They're all connected!

Even more disturbing is the fact that shoulder pain is one of the most difficult conditions to treat. When you fall or strain your shoulder, the resulting pushing and pulling forces cause injury to the neck and shoulder bones. These displacements cause pressure on the nerves and blood vessels, diminishing their abilities to heal themselves. Muscles then become unbalanced. Stronger muscles then push or pull abnormally hard against the weaker ones, and if not treated, shoulder problems may progress to an extremely painful and limiting condition called tendonitis.

Chiropractic doctors are experts at finding and treating these types of problems. With the proper adjustments, the pain, numbness, and tingling can be brought under control; not only in the shoulder, but in the neck, arm, wrist, and hands as well.

## OTHER PAIN RELIEVABLE BY CHIROPRACTIC CARE

The fact that everything is connected is apparent in the many different causes of pain that can be treated by an adjustment of the spine. I bet you never considered going to the chiropractor to relieve that jaw, leg, or finger pain, did you?

### Sciatica

"My leg hurts."

Is that sciatic pain? Or did you run into the door this morning when you got out of bed? What does leg pain mean? Well, other than the fact that your leg hurts, it can mean a lot of things. Not *all* leg pain is sciatica, but sciatica usually causes pain in the leg, or worse yet, both legs.

The sciatic nerve is another good example of the way parts of our bodies are connected and how each individual part affects the next one, and the next one, and so on. It is made up of five nerves that leave the spinal cord from the lower spinal column, join in the pelvic area, and then travel down the leg where they divide into many smaller nerves that reach the muscles and joints of the thigh, knee, calf, ankle, feet, and toes. The sciatic nerve is the longest and largest nerve in the body. Those who suffer from severe pain along the sciatic nerve path can tell you without reservation that they hurt all over.

*Sciatica* is a problem that begins in the spine, but symptoms often appear in the legs first. The pain of sciatica, which is caused by inflammation of the sciatic nerve, is sometimes described as a "pins and needles" feeling, and often is accompanied by tenderness; sharp pain; burning, tingling, prickling, or crawling sensations; and numbness. The location of the pain varies from the back of the legs and thighs, to the ankles, feet, and toes. Some individuals also complain of pain in the front or side of their legs, as well as in the hips. Duration of the pain ranges from a constant throbbing, which may last several days, to quick, sharp stabs, sometimes brought about by simply standing up or lying down. Some poor souls even have *bi-lateral sciatica*, which means both legs are affected. In severe cases, sciatica can cause a wasting of the calf muscles or a loss of reflexes.

The cause of sciatica is a little less complex than the cause of some of the other ailments we've discussed in this chapter. It can be caused by a misalignment in the spine or a pro-truded or ruptured disc irritating the sciatic nerve. Arthritis of the spine can cause sciatic pain, as can constipation, tumors, or even vitamin deficiencies. Although back or hip problems may often occur before sciatica symptoms appear, there are times when it happens without any prior announcement from any of the other areas of the body. Like the lower back, it takes a lot to hurt the sciatic nerve, but once it is injured, it takes a lot to heal it.

## Neurogenic Claudication

If the spinal nerves that go to the legs become damaged, it can cause a condition known as *neurogenic claudication*. I doubt that you will ever hear anyone at the mall say they have to stop walking for a while because of neurogenic claudication, because many have never even heard of it. Neurogenic claudication is leg pain caused by poor blood circulation due to nerve dam-age. What this means for the sufferer, in plain English, is that the person cannot walk for long periods of time without stop-ping to rest because of pain, cramping, numbness, aching, and fatigue, usually in the calf, although it can also appear in the foot, thigh, hip, or buttocks.

Medical treatments for neurogenic claudication may include painkillers, muscle relaxants, and various orthopedic treatments including physical therapy and traction. Sometimes the pain may become so intense that even strong painkilling drugs bring little relief to the sufferer. This severe condition may require painkilling drugs to be injected directly into the nerve roots to bring relief to the patient. This, of course, can cause dependency upon the strong medication. Patients who suffer from these se-vere symptoms are often advised to have surgery.

Again, I cannot stress enough that the chiropractic alternative could help avoid this surgery and should be tried first before any medical or surgical procedures are undertaken. Regular chiropractic treatment keeps the nervous system free of any interference and will help prevent conditions like neurogenic claudication.

## Temporomandibular Joint Disorder (TMJ)

The temporomandibular joint is formed by the temporal (a skull bone) and the mandible (the lower jawbone). If you place your fingers in front of your ear, you can feel the temporomandibular joint when you open or close your mouth. Doesn't seem as though it could cause too much trouble, does it? Guess again. When this area becomes dysfunctional, your problems multiply in a big hurry. Not only is it extremely painful, it is a source of many other problems (isn't everything connected?), such as headaches and neck and back pain. Sometimes it can cause other difficulties seemingly unrelated to the jaw joint such as nervousness, emotional problems, loss of balance, anxiety, high blood pressure, nausea, visual disturbance, dizziness, hearing loss, speech lisps, and even shoulder pain.

All this from a small space in front of your ear?

It's all connected.

I have stressed many times in this book the importance of medical and chiropractic doctors working together for the good of the patient. Temporomandibular joint disorder (TMJ) often requires the services of the family dentist, orthodontist, and chiropractor. Sometimes one of them may be able to correct the problem (with time), but the ideal situation is for all of them to work together.

Dentists, orthodontists, and chiropractors know the number of problems associated with TMJ, as well as the various causes. Malocclusion of the teeth can be one cause of TMJ, as can various injuries and muscle imbalance. Even some children who lay on the floor to read or watch television with their chins propped up in their hands can develop this condition. A little slap on the chin may not seem much at the time, but weeks, even months later, you may find yourself suffering from TMJ. Stress is also a big factor in TMJ problems. No one will have to tell you that you have a problem. If the pain itself were not enough, the inability to open your jaw more than the space of a quarter inch or less, is a sure sign. There is usually a clicking or popping sound when the jaw opens as well. Soreness of the joint while chewing can be another sign that something is amiss.

TMJ is not a problem to take lightly, especially since there is a close connection between the temporomandibular joint and the nerve communication from the brain, which in turn can affect many other body parts and functions. Chiropractors help people every day with TMJ. That's right. Amazingly, an adjustment to the spine even helps relieve problems in the jaw. We treat them with adjustments and specific exercises, eliminating the cause of the symptoms. As in other cases, surgery should be a last resort. In my office, I have had great results with TMJ sufferers.

## Carpal Tunnel Syndrome (CTS)

Isn't it amazing how a condition you've never heard of suddenly becomes the "problem of the year" for everybody? You hear of one person who has it, then everybody has carpal tunnel syndrome.

It is believed by some medical authorities that carpal tunnel syndrome (CTS) may affect one out of ten Americans who work with their hands; especially those who engage in repetitive tasks, such as secretaries, assembly line workers, and professional drivers.

Recently, there has been a rash of carpal tunnel syndrome diagnoses. It is a little like flying saucers—one sighting and everybody's seen one. It has become an increasingly costly problem, not only to those who suffer from it, but for businesses and industries, due to missed work by employees.

What is a carpal tunnel? Is it on the Pennsylvania Turnpike?

Actually, the carpal tunnel is formed by the wrist (carpal) bones, which form a tunnel-like structure through which pass nine tendons and the median nerve. Carpal tunnel syndrome occurs when the median nerve is pinched or pressured. Sometimes a medical doctor will try to relieve the pain by using a splint to immobilize the wrist and prescribing diuretics (which decrease water build-up and swelling) or anti-inflammatory drugs, or by suggesting the use of ice packs. Corticosteroids are sometimes injected into the crease of the hand near the wrist and may provide some temporary relief. The pain usually returns, however, and the side effects from the medication can be quite severe.

The final resort, medically speaking, is surgery, from which recovery may take from six months to ten years. Say again? *Six months to ten years*—or never. This unsatisfactory medical treatment prompted the late Robert Mendelsohn, M.D., to recommend that his patients consult experts in muscle and joint therapy for CTS.

Alternatives to surgery for this condition are exercises, soft tissue therapy, and physical therapy. It has also been noted that certain nutritional supplements such as vitamin $B_6$ have been shown to be effective for patients with this condition.

Anyone suffering from CTS should consult with a chiropractor to ensure that the spine is free from nerve stress and nerve impingement, since there is a direct connection between arm and wrist pain and the nerves that come from the neck. One controlled clinical study of CTS sufferers found that after chiropractic care, improvements were demonstrated in all strength and range of motion measures.

## "IT'S TOO QUIET OUT THERE, I DON'T LIKE IT."

Your body gives you a number of signals trying to warn you that there is trouble when there is a problem with your spine. These signals should be heeded immediately, not ignored. Do you think for one minute that John Wayne would have ignored a series of smoke signals while riding through hostile territory? Would he have just ridden on through the pass without checking it out?

Nobody wants to ride into an ambush of serious disease or deterioration, especially when you've had fair warning signs by the nagging pain in the lower part of your back. The following are just a few of the symptoms you need to look for to be able to head off a more serious problem:

- Mild, nagging discomfort in the lower back.
- Pain or numbness in the legs and/or feet.
- Hemorrhoids.

- Swelling of the ankles.
- Fatigue in the lower back.
- Kidney or bladder disorders.
- Blemishes on your skin.
- Stomach disorders.
- Constipation or recurring diarrhea.
- Menstrual problems.
- Sterility.
- Impotence or prostate problems.
- Pain while sitting for extended periods.

If you have any of these symptoms, they may be smoke signals that there are very serious problems ahead. To proceed through the unguarded canyon without concern could very well cause you a great deal of woe.

And we all hate *woe*, don't we?

## LESS IS MORE

By the time most people decide to do something about their back pain, they usually go to a medical doctor who prescribes medication or may recommend surgery as treatment for their back problems. Surgery is not always necessary. Your chiropractor can provide a painless, effective alternative to surgery.

The sad part for most back surgery patients is that back surgery has been called one of the most unnecessarily performed surgical procedures in medicine today. To add insult to injury, it is successful only about 50 percent of the time. There are approximately 600,000 back surgeries performed every year (and the number is growing) and this leaves 300,000 back pain sufferers still looking for different answers.

The unfortunate thing is that most people don't seek chiropractic help for their back problems, even though it has been proven again and again that chiropractors know how to take care of your pain. They'll go to a medical doctor or osteopath first, where they are given drugs and are told to apply heat to the area and get plenty of rest.

---

# *Did You Know...*

... that the largest health maintenance organization in the southeastern United States, AV MED, recently conducted an impressive study? Twelve patients who were medically diagnosed as needing disc surgery were sent to a chiropractor who corrected all twelve of the cases, saving the HMO $250,000 in surgical costs. Dr. Herbert Davis, M.D., medical director of AV MED and author of the study, admitted to being a skeptic initially but said that the study proved "to be a real eye-opening experience on the effectiveness of chiropractic."

... that another important conclusion was made by the RAND study in Santa Monica, California in 1991? This think tank, an internationally known and highly respected non-profit research corporation, conducted an exhaustive evaluation of scientific literature. The panel of experts, which included neurologists, medical orthopedists, and chiropractors, came to the conclusion that spinal manipulation, as used by chiropractors, is an effective and appropriate treatment for low-back disorders.

---

Sometimes, if the problem is not too severe, the body can help itself under these circumstances for a while at least. But the underlying problem (subluxation) is still there. By the time you seek chiropractic care when the drugs no longer work, your problem will be much worse due to age and deterioration. Chiropractors rarely get the easy problems. Normally, we get the most difficult, chronic, painful problems of weakened backs—then get complaints about how long it takes to fix something that has been "broken" for so long. I can't begin to count how many times I've had people come into my office and say to me that they've been every place else, and I am their last hope.

Think of chiropractic *first*!

According to one study of 1,536 lumbar spinal problem patients who were under chiropractic care, 96.4 percent had satisfactory results. Only 3.6 percent of the patients turned to surgery. I would call those very impressive numbers.

Chiropractors work with the spine. If you have back pain or pain related to the back, it makes sense that you should go to someone who treats the back. You should seek chiropractic help at *the first sign* of a problem, not as a last resort. The sooner you get a diagnosis of your problem and begin treatment, the better. Most people wait too long to begin proper care.

"Back pain sufferers who take less medication and move around a lot will recover just as well as people told to take more medicine and rest."

Is this your chiropractor talking?

No. This is the conclusion of a 1994 study done by the Center of Heath Studies and the University of Washington in Seattle. Isn't that what I've been telling you? Isn't that what chiropractic teaches?

News flash! The study showed that patients given the least medical attention were more satisfied with their treatment and were charged 79-percent less than whose who were medicated. If less is just as good (medically speaking) in the treatment of back pain, then why do we take more medicine for it?

Because our doctor says it will help us?

Because we want to kill that pain—at any cost?

Because we don't know what else to do?

All of the above?

That everything is connected within our body is an undisputed fact. Nothing in our bodies is an island unto itself. Since everything is connected, one problem can lead to another and another until the entire body is in jeopardy. Chapters 7 and 8 discuss the many illnesses that can occur due to misalignment of the spine. The good news is that a spinal adjustment can also correct whatever is connected to the spine, and so on, and so on. The trick here is to keep the main line (spine) healthy, and the rest of the body will most likely fall into the line marked "Good Health."

If we recall the old gospel song about "Them Bones," we will recall that the hip bone is connected to the thigh bone, the thigh bone is connected to the knee bone, and so on, ending with "and the bones got up and they walked around. . . ."

Some people with bad backs wish they could do as well.

# Chapter 5

# Life Is Neutral
## (So Is Your All-Important Immune System)

*The soldiers had been fighting on an island for several weeks. They were down to only three men, and they knew their chances were indeed slim. The enemy was attacking from the sea, and behind them lay the dark and dense jungle.*

*"There's no use in trying to escape through that dangerous jungle," one said. "It is a far worse fate than the enemy, with all the snakes, wild animals, and quicksand. We'll never come out alive. The jungle is a killer."*

*A second man, with a shudder, agreed.*

*The third looked in front of him at his fierce enemy, then behind him at the jungle. He wondered if they could be wrong.*

*When the first man who had spoken was taken down by a bullet, the second one raised his hands in surrender and walked out on to the beach. The last man looked back at the jungle and wondered if it would really kill him. He knew the enemy would. Suddenly, amid a hail of bullets, he made a run for it. The enemy did not bother to chase him, for they, too, believed the jungle would devour him.*

*He was trembling with fear, and his heart pounded as he made his way into the thick undergrowth. He could hear sounds and movement, but he kept running. Soon, he found himself deep inside the jungle. He stopped and looked around. He could still hear the sounds all about him, and he knew he was now part of the jungle.*

*His fears subsided somewhat. As the hours went by, he became less and less frightened, and before long he made an amazing discovery. The jungle was not his enemy. It was not out to kill him or to do him any harm whatsoever.*

*However, he also made another startling discovery. The jungle was also not out to help him. He was on his own. The jungle was absolutely neutral.*

*So is life. Life is neutral.*

Your immune system is also neutral. It can help you—or it can work against you. It is not out to kill you, although it can. It is not out to save you, although it can do that as well. You are on your own. If you take care of your immune system, it will protect you because, basically, that is the way our creator designed it. Even though it can and does attack you at times, it has no particular grudge against you. It does not get angry and turn on you like a vicious animal might. It does not use any extra energy to do anything beyond what it was designed to do. The bottom line is that your immune system will work for you—if you will work with it.

The ancient philosopher Lao-tzu wrote thousands of years ago, "Nature is extremely impartial." According to Biblical ideology we are all viewed without preference. Since the immune system is part of our nature, we have to understand its impartiality as well. We also know that the immune system is one of the most amazing things about a living, breathing human being. We are told in the first chapter of the Bible (Genesis 1:26–27) that we were created in God's image. I don't believe this image is one of sickness, pain, and disease. I do believe we have everything within ourselves to maintain our bodies, to be strong and healthy, and to die of natural causes at a very, very old age.

What we do know about our bodies' immune systems is quite amazing and wonderful. At its best the system will keep you safe from disease. The immune system, when healthy and working the way it was designed, labors without ceasing to keep you in good health. Much like an elite patrol guard (although much less expensive and more dependable) it can search out each and every bacterial virus and every other microorganism or dangerous invader and destroy them like a Batman comic. ZAP! BAAM! WHAM!

This amazing protector gets rid of anything that is not supposed to be in our systems. Unhampered by sentiments, ego, or choices, it takes no prisoners. Like our modern-day computers, it even has a memory and can recall old battle plans for a more immediate response to new encounters with old enemies. Today's modern warfare has "smart" missiles, but they are nothing compared to the way our immune systems can zero in on a target and destroy it. What a great friend to have on your side!

However, as pointed out before, the immune system is neither friend nor foe. It is simply doing its job. That is, if all is well. And if it isn't? Well, just as it can save your life, it can take it. It can also stand by and allow something else to take it, or—worst case scenario—it can attack you itself right along with the invader in your body. That is an awesome power this system holds over you. It can be both comforting and frightening. The same power the system uses daily to keep you from falling victim to some dreaded disease can go haywire and, not only fail to protect you, but actually turn its guns on you from within, crippling your good cells and allowing the bad ones to have their way with you.

Horror story? Sometimes. But we are not without some control over our bodies' complex systems.

## HOW THE IMMUNE SYSTEM WORKS

We have a number of weapons to protect us from external threats to our bodies' good health—the most notable one being the skin, which creates that first barrier to dangerous invaders. This layer of important protective tissue is not even 1/20 of an inch thick, yet it is a highly effective barrier to most *pathogens* (anything capable of causing disease). Not only that, but the acidic nature of sweat and other sebaceous gland secretions on the body's surface can also be toxic, thus helping to repel fungi and bacteria.

If you've ever wondered why we have those tiny hairs inside our noses—they certainly do not enhance our looks—they serve a very good purpose. They are effective in trapping fairly large particles that could prove detrimental to our health—and I'll do you a favor by not going into any further description at this point. Another deterrent to those "enemies" is mucus, which forms a fluid physical barrier that traps particulate matter and keeps it from invading the underlying cells. The mucus is then moved away from the cell surface through the sweeping activity of the protective hairlike projections, called the *cilia*, that line the bronchial passageways. The mucous membranes lining the respiratory and digestive tracts are active in the first line of defense. Any inhaled or ingested pathogen must pass through the mucous membrane defenses before it can do any damage inside the body. There are also *macrophages* in the lungs and bronchial region that swallow up pathogens that have become trapped in the mucus. Does all this sound a bit boring and technical? Okay, let's get a bit more graphic. It's not really a dinner table subject, but when the mucus is expelled, it is gone from our system. This is the way we get rid of a lot of germs. Even if it is swallowed, the digestive tract takes over its job and proves hostile (and usually fatal) to these pesky little invaders. The throat and esophagus provide little protection, but stomach fluid is high in acid and destroys any microorganism it encounters in its territory.

If, however, the invaders get past this area—primarily due to poorly chewed or undercooked food—and the acid does not reach them, then problems do occur. This might be a good place to point out that "mother did know best" when she told you again and again to chew your food well. This is not only essential for digestion (and good manners), but for the protection against disease as well.

What happens if a pathogen has managed to get through the nose or the mouth and past the stomach? Picture the little critter jumping up and down and yelling "home free!" It has now reached an area where growth can take place. It can thrive in this area because the intestines, in a healthy digestive system, are already occupied with a heavy concentration of bacteria that are either neutral or beneficial.

The new kid is not going to have it easy, however. The newly arrived organism is at a distinct disadvantage when competing for resources. Some of the resident bacteria also produce antibiotic-like substances as part of their by-products, making the environment even more difficult for the intruder.

The harmful effects of smoking are important to consider in the immune system as well. Smoking damages both the cilia and the macrophages in the lungs, causing the physical defenses to break down and fail to protect you against disease. In short, it is yet another gate left open for the dangerous invaders to sneak through.

And crying doesn't help. . . . Well, yes, it does. Lysozyme is found in large quantities in our tears. Our eyes are protected through their constant washing by tears—even when we're not crying. The teardrops are transported through a duct into the back of the throat, where pathogens are subject to the digestive system defense team. See how wonderfully designed we are! Even tears have a purpose—other than the obvious ones used by children or a sweetheart to help convince someone to give them sympathy, comfort, or aid.

The body has many other ways to protect itself. Fevers are part of our defense mechanism. They burn off microorganisms. Swelling is another helpful advantage. It helps wash the system by bringing fluids to the injured area (which causes the swelling). The fluid helps take away debris, germs, and bacteria that may have invaded the area. Swelling also reduces movement, thus protecting the area. We also have cells that attack and devour intruders—T cells, killer cells, lymphocytes, antibodies, antitoxins, interferon, and other cells and chemicals, each with its own little job to do. Talk about your busy bodies. Ours certainly are, for which we can be eternally thankful.

If the body suffers a puncture wound, a pathogen can just jump right in there and begin its journey to whatever area it can do the most harm—that is, if our defenses are down and fail to zap the critter in its tracks.

At the risk of sounding like an excerpt from a children's story, let us look at this whole thing from a whimsical point of view. Sometimes things can get a bit too technical.

### Sammy Splinter, the Bad Guy

Sammy Splinter has attacked you, and before you can do anything about it, he and his germ-laden body (and possibly some of his cruddy soldiers) are seeking to invade the cavity made when you stepped on that old splintered wooden board on the boat dock.

Sammy and his accomplices are inside now, happy that they

have indeed gotten past that first line of defense—the skin—that usually protects you from the initial invaders. And let's say that you even manage to extract Sammy from the skin's edge early on, his dirty little accomplices—dirt, germs, etc.—may still remain, working their way into your system seeking something to infect and destroy. Once inside, however, evil Sammy and his friends find there are still many obstacles to overcome.

They are very discouraged to discover that most of your internal organs are surrounded by a tough membranous capsule, which is even more resistant to penetration than the organ tissue it protects. Sammy and his cronies will have much difficulty here.

Next, the little band of no-gooders may encounter *macromolecules*, which are very large chain-like molecules in the blood that have antibacterial or antiviral properties. One of these molecules, called *glycoproteins*, may surround this mangy little group and prevent them from reaching a target cell and causing infestation. ("Curses, foiled again!") Doesn't all this sound exciting? Three cheers for the good guys! In addition, there are iron-bearing protein molecules in the blood that compete with bacteria for the iron required for growth and reproduction. You'd think these little ruffians would not have a chance—but they are never to be underestimated. Even though our good friends, the B and T cells, which constantly roam the body seeking invaders to kill, sometimes fail to "head 'em off at the pass," you can rest assured that they will do their level best.

Let's say for the purpose of a happy ending that Sammy's little band of meanies lose this battle. They are reduced to spit and left on the ground to die. Perhaps they were (Gasp!) flushed down the toilet. Either way, they are gone from the system that has fought so valiantly for your good health. The good guys have won!

Fairy tale? Fiction? Magic? No, it's reality. It's nature's way of doing business. We have a great little group of fighters inside all of us, and that's not all. We have an internal defense industry made up of hard-working and loyal organs that produce the weapons to be used against these invaders. Our bone marrow, spleen, thymus, adenoids, appendix, and lymph nodes all must remain healthy to give us lots of high-quality armaments for this constant battle.

## Natural Immunity

Our immune systems are incredibly sophisticated and complicated parts of us, by which our bodies are able to naturally resist disease and infection. Natural immunity begins when we
are conceived. Unfortunately, some diseases can be transmitted
from mother to child in the birth canal. This is why expectant
mothers must take exceptional care of themselves, giving the
baby the best possible chance for good health from the beginning. Drugs and chemicals (including alcohol, tobacco, caffeine,
and even artificial sweeteners) cross the placenta as well—hence
the importance of the expectant mother following a good and
healthy diet. Besides, there is certainly nothing wrong with the
mother being in the best possible health in order to enjoy and
care for this newborn treasure.

There are two schools of thought about how large a part the
mother plays in the overall immunity of the child she carries.
One, the *germline theory,* is that an infant inherits all of his or
her antibodies genetically from the parents. The second theory,
the *somatic mutation theory,* holds that the mother passes on only
a few antibodies—genetically through the placenta, as well as
through her milk—which then mutate into all the rest.

When we talk about the immune system, it is unfortunate
that the constitution declaring that "all men (and women) are
created equal" does not continue to apply. Even if we were all
created equal—and if proper prenatal care were universal, perhaps we would be—but the fact is, we certainly do not remain
equal when it comes to our good health. There are several mod-
ifying factors that can influence the effectiveness of the body's
defenses. There are many things that go into the making of a
healthy and effective immune system.

It has been proven that breast-fed babies have fewer illnesses (infections, allergies, colds, etc.) than those who are bottle-
fed. Plus, there is the added bonus for the nursing mother, who
has less chance of developing breast cancer later in life. It's no
wonder that some parents become confused at the mixed messages coming from the medical profession, but rest assured that
mother's milk contains lifesaving antibodies not found in cow,
goat, or soybean milk.

Hey, I'm sorry, but I just don't believe people can duplicate nature. I'm also sorry to say that many people think they can improve on nature, but the simple truth is that if you want to have the healthiest baby possible—breast-feed! You will be raising a healthier baby who will grow into a healthier adult.

## WHAT CAN GO WRONG
## IN THE IMMUNE SYSTEM

An unhealthy immune system can sweep through your body like a roaring lion, devouring all of your defenses. It can overreact in its protection when it attacks foreign objects, which is what happens to those who are *allergic* or *hypersensitive*. It can underreact and fail to defend the body, which is called an *immunologic deficiency disorder*. And the worst horror story is when it attacks the body it was meant to serve (*autoimmune disorders*).

Most are familiar with the story of the "Boy in the Bubble." It was made into a television movie and was the subject of several documentaries and articles in newspapers, magazines, and medical journals. The boy, who was born with no immune system, lived all his short life in a specially controlled, germ-free "plastic bubble" in a hospital room in Houston, Texas. He breathed filtered air from which any bacteria, viruses, and any other foreign substances were removed. Even his food had to be sterilized and introduced to him through air locks. He was not able to leave his plastic bubble even for normal family interactions, including hugs and kisses, until after receiving a bone marrow transplant at the age of 12. Unfortunately, the boy died that same year, as a result of complications following the transplant. That is the longest life span on record for anyone born without a functioning immune system. Babies born with this disability seldom make it through the first year.

This story is an amazing example of the immune system and what it means to our bodies. Millions of dollars and equipment, plus countless hours of devotion from doctors and family could only prolong the inevitable death of the child. We cannot survive or live a normal life without our immune systems. This story only underscores the seeming simplicity of the way our immune system works when it is normal, and the complications (and death) it can cause when it is not.

Do we know why the external and internal defense forces

do not function at the same level of efficiency in all individuals?

As is the case with much of health care, we don't know all the reasons, but we do know many of them. It is generally recognized that such factors as race, sex, nutritional health, hormonal influences, fatigue, climate, age, stress, traumatic injury, radiation, drug use, and alcoholism greatly influence the level of a person's natural resistance—which is your natural immune system. In all of the immune-related disorders, the white blood cells and their functions may be greatly inhibited by a number of these factors.

Take the common cold—as Rodney Dangerfield so aptly puts it—*please!* We will all agree that the way the common cold makes us feel is anything but common. Has the medical profession, with all its resources and billions of dollars, managed to cure—or even come close to curing—the common cold? Of course not.

In order to produce the symptoms we recognize as a cold— sore throat, runny nose, cough, sneezing, and a general all-over case of the "miseries"—it takes one or more of more than 100 different strains of viruses. Your system may be prepared to repel only fifty different types, and guess what? The virus with which you come in contact is one of the *other* fifty, causing you to fall victim to this most aggravating of maladies.

What it all comes down to is very simple. If your immune system is in good working order, you may not even notice the few sniffles before they disappear. You may recall times when you *thought* you were coming down with a cold, but nothing really happened, and the following day you felt fine. Your immune system was in top form and did its job. If it had not been working properly, you would have spent several days in discomfort, not to mention the discomfort you may have caused everyone with whom you came in contact, whether by passing on your little "germ," or simply by driving them crazy with your coughing, sneezing, sniffling, and whining.

## THE MEDICAL APPROACH
## TO THE IMMUNE SYSTEM

Medical doctors know a lot about tne immune system. They are acutely aware of its functions and its malfunctions. But again, the problem with today's medicine—a problem acknowledged by most medical educators and practicing physicians alike—is that theirs is a *reactive* approach to health. Few medical doctors really believe in the body's ability to heal itself. They really don't believe the body can be well without interference. They believe in medical *intervention.* They think that they know more than the body does. They do not focus on the *prevention* of illness, which our immune system can help us accomplish. Modern medicine, with all its pharmaceutical weapons, is not even called into the picture until there is a disease to fight. Only then does medicine hone in on the target. By this time, unfortunately, it is often too late.

Most medical doctors believe the body is going to break down, get sick, or become diseased, and they will fix it. This is the way they treat their patients, family, friends, and colleagues. They test each other, drug each other, and perform surgeries on each other because their professional ideals are based on disease *treatment,* not disease *prevention.* And those people who do nothing to prevent illness and disease will need to keep in very close contact with their medical doctors because they will, for a fact, need their services.

## A Trip to the Doctor

Imagine this little scenario the next time you visit your family medical doctor: The doctor walks into the examining room where you've been waiting for thirty minutes (after an hour and fifteen minutes in the waiting room) and asks you how you are.

"I'm just fine, thank you," you reply.

"You feel *fine*?" She sounds a bit perplexed.

"Yes, I do."

"Well, then what are you *doing* here?" She is beginning to sound irritated. She doesn't have time for her patients to come in just to tell her they are feeling fine.

"Because I want to feel fine in the future. I *like* feeling fine."

What do you suppose the doctor says now? Is she going to call a mental institution and have you committed—she'd probably like to—or is she going to smile pleasantly, tell you to keep doing whatever it is you're doing, dismiss you, and send a bill for $48?

If a person has no symptoms, the medical doctor doesn't know what to do. Actually, it's not his or her job to do anything for well people. They are "sick" doctors, not "well" doctors. That's not a criticism—*it's the way things are.* Well, OK, maybe it *is* a criticism—but it's still *the way things are.*

My question to you now is this: The man who suffered a heart attack on Monday—was he *healthy* on Sunday? Even though he had no symptoms on Sunday—felt good, as a matter fact—laughed and played golf. Was he *really* healthy? I don't think so.

Take the woman who notices a frightening nodule in her breast on Friday. Was she well on Thursday? Did this happen overnight? We know it did not. The little boy who was out happily playing with his friends on Tuesday develops a terrible cold on Wednesday. Was he healthy on Tuesday? Did this happen overnight? We know it did not. We may have believed he was healthy on Tuesday, but in truth, he was not.

The aforementioned three people were not healthy the day before they got sick. They may have had no symptoms, but they were *not* healthy. We suffer under the dangerous delusion that if we have no symptoms or we have no disease, then we are well!

What I'm saying—and continue to repeat again and again and again—is that the best way to be healthy is to stay well. The best way to stay well is not to get sick. Oh sure, you say, those are only words. No, it makes a lot more sense than you might think. In order to keep from getting sick, you must begin to understand how your body works, and take care of it regularly, not just when you have symptoms as organized medicine would have us believe you should. As we age, we should take better care of ourselves, but, unfortunately, we do not. In fact, many people take *less* care of themselves as they get older. There is a great push now for proper diet and exercise. Health clubs are everywhere, and who do you find there? Right, it's the younger people, and that's good. That's good, *if* they keep it up and even increase it as they get older.

We, and by we I mean *all the American people,* have actually been brainwashed into believing that what the medical profession offers us is health care. If you've read this far, you know that I do not consider it health care at all, but *sick care!*

## The Search for Cures

How many *billions* of dollars have Americans spent on research—looking for cancer cures, diabetes cures, arthritis cures, and all kinds of other cures? We have some very caring and dedicated people working late into the nights in lonely laboratories all over the country. We have more caring people going from door to door looking for donations from other caring, well-meaning people. We collect funds for the relief of heart diseases, kidney ailments, diabetes, cancer, AIDS, and any number of terrible and sometimes deadly diseases. We have Jerry's kids, telethons, marathons, ugly bartender contests, hiking, biking, and every other type of fund-raising effort in attempts to find a cure or some relief for these diseases that beset and sometimes destroy us. What has to become *painfully* clear to us is this:

There are no cures.

There are no cures.

*There are no cures.*

What have we cured? Heart problems? No. Diabetes? No. Hypertension? No. Arthritis? No. The common cold? No. The flu? No. Cancer? No. Polio? No. Even with the vaccine, it is not cured.

The list goes on and on, but *there are no cures*. There can be temporary relief. There may even be some remissions, but there are no cures. In fact, there are more new diseases now than ever—for which we also have no cure. There is, however, a ray of hope. There *are* preventions.

A few years ago, a 23-year-old woman came into my office with back pain. As we were going over her medical history, I discovered she'd had her gallbladder removed, but had not written down that she had gallbladder problems on the form my new patients fill out.

When I asked why, she said, "Oh, I'm cured of my gallbladder problems."

I asked her how she was cured.

She looked at me as though I was stupid. "Because it's gone. I don't *have* it," she said curtly, "therefore, it's not a problem. It's *cured*." I was sitting there wondering how in the logical world does taking out your gallbladder heal it. That doesn't heal it. You can cut the thing out, but it's still a sick gallbladder. It's the same for the removal of tonsils or other organs. They are not *cured* just because they are *gone.*

"You're 23 years old, and you don't have a gallbladder," I said, "and you seem quite happy about it." She glared at me. I then went on to tell her that actually *curing* her gallbladder would mean finding out what was wrong, what caused it to malfunction, then fix the malfunction so the gallbladder would work the way it was meant to work in the first place.

"You need a gallbladder to help break down fat," I said. "After all, the gallbladder stores bile that helps the body break down fat." Whatever nerve interference caused her gallbladder to go bad at age 23, could still be doing damage to her body in other places now that the gallbladder is gone. Still, she felt she was *cured.* I was glad she hadn't gone to her doctor for a severe headache.

Brainwashed people of the world—*wake up!*

It wasn't too long ago that physicians actually used x-rays to kill the thymus gland in young children because it was larger than they thought it should be. I'm sure many of you still remember this procedure. Since our bodies are made to be perfect in the beginning, there was a good reason for the larger size of the thymus gland in children. It was put there to help fight off infection and disease that is so prevalent in those tender years. Even though medical doctors no longer do this as a routine procedure, I have to wonder how many children were needlessly hurt because of it. How many lives were shortened due to their medical intervention?

Another routine procedure when I was a kid, was the removal of a child's tonsils and adenoids. Chiropractors were against this, even then, because they knew that God didn't make a mistake and put in something that our bodies didn't need. Taking out the tonsils and adenoids (unless they are in terrible shape) is rarely done these days, so perhaps progress is being made. However, the medical community has progressed to other popular procedures such as the insertion of tubes in the ears as a treatment for chronic ear infections, drugs for hyperactivity, and antibiotics for just about everything else. We ought to ask ourselves how many of these procedures in years to come will prove to be ineffective and even dangerous to the young patients.

## Drugs

While some reasonably healthy people do go to their doctors for a yearly checkup, even if they feel fine, most people go to a medical doctor or a chiropractor only when they can't stand the pain any longer. By then their natural defenses are fighting, or have already fought the illness, and may very well be losing. There are five danger words we should always watch out for: "Maybe it will go away."

If we go to a medical doctor, what are we going to get? It will be one of three things: tests, drugs, or surgery—maybe all three.

Some people have terrible reactions to various drugs. Others are hurt more than they are helped. Granted, some drugs have saved lives. Unfortunately, some "cures" have caused death.

What many people don't know is that antibiotics don't kill viruses. Did you know that? Furthermore, antibiotics are not only *not* helpful in fighting viral infections, but are actually detrimental to the body's natural ability to regain health. Medicines such as tetracycline, sulfa drugs, penicillin, and many others fight bacteria one way or another. Some also combat microorganisms that have characteristics of both viruses and bacteria, as well as fungi (molds, mildew, growths) and protozoa (microscopic, one-celled organisms). Even the few antiviral drugs that do exist have potentially damaging side effects because they are toxic to body cells. Viruses live within the body's cells, depending on the cells' metabolism for reproduction, and the only way to fight them chemically is by attacking the very cells they infest. It is a little like burning down the house to get rid of the roaches—effective on one hand, but hardly a solution if you ever want to live in the house again. The overuse of antibiotics has become very dangerous, since organisms that are resistant to the types of antibiotics prescribed can multiply when competing microorganisms, killed by antibiotics, are removed.

And what will happen when the medical profession begins to realize that these drugs no longer work and have been overprescribed? This is already a reality. Antibiotics as we know them will soon become a thing of the past because of their inability to fight new strains of antibiotic-resistant bacteria, strange new germs, and out-of-control viruses.

When antibiotics were introduced as "the answer" to many illnesses after World War II, there was much optimism in both the medical community and the general public. Soon, it was believed, there would be an end to many of the major illnesses. The unlimited promises held by such drugs as penicillin, sulfa drugs, and a number of other antibiotics, seemed to be the hoped-and-prayed-for miracles to wipe out infection, save lives, and eradicate infections forever. To say that some of these antibiotics have not been of certain value in fighting various illnesses would not be true, but at what price? And has the result been what we had all hoped it would be?

When the country's surgeon general told Congress twenty-five years ago that it was time to "close the book on infectious disease," there was understandably a great collective sigh of relief from the health-conscious population. We had finally licked these dreaded diseases! Or had we?

In the last two decades, dangerous infectious diseases have made a dramatic and frightening comeback! Furthermore, they are stronger than ever in their attacks. We are not only facing new and more deadly "monsters," but those we thought we had defeated have come back to taunt us, each one finding new ways to outwit the "cures."

What's even worse, is that some common bacteria, such as streptococcus, have produced rare, virulent strains capable of killing in a matter of days. The tale of the so-called "flesh-eating" bacteria is the kind of story the tabloids thrive on. Unfortunately, the horror stories are a reasonably accurate account of this "new" strain of infection.

## Who or What Has Unleashed These Monsters Upon Us?

There is no single Pandora who has opened the "box of troubles." We have always had plagues and diseases—just as we have always had resources to fight them. The experts tell us that there are several reasons for the more recent resurgence of infectious diseases.

1. The use and misuse of antibiotics, which has allowed rapidly reproducing bacteria to adapt and mutate into strains that

# *Did You Know...*

... Life gets more treacherous every day. This may sound like something out of a horror movie or a Robin Cook novel, but, unfortunately, it is fact!

The August 22, 1997 edition of the *Akron Beacon Journal* reported that a staph germ that is showing resistance to medicine's "drug of last resort" has appeared for the first time in the United States. A new strain of *staphylococcus aureus* bacteria was found in a Michigan man suffering from kidney failure. The patient had a recurring infection where the catheter for dialysis was inserted. He was being treated with vancomycin, the antibiotic that has always been successfully used to fight infection when all else failed since 1970, when the bacteria began showing resistance to the drug. He is currently being treated with a combination of drugs, including vancomycin, but it can only be a matter of time until the infection starts resisting this treatment as well.

Since the introduction of penicillin in the early 1950s (then touted as a "cure-all"), chiropractors have tried to warn the general public about the dangers of antibiotics. While lives have been saved by antibiotics, they are not a cure-all and never will be. Antibiotics have been overused from their inception, and it was just a matter of time before some new frightening, antibiotic-resistant strain appeared.

are resistant to any conventional treatment. In my opinion, this is the main reason for the resurgence of infectious diseases.

2. The changing dynamics of our societies today—from the urbanization of the Third World to modern intercontinental air travel—which allows for the rapid transmission of disease from country to country.

3. The destruction of many ecosystems, including tropical rain forests and jungles, has toyed with nature's balance and destroyed many natural healing properties that are found in these areas. Furthermore, it has placed people in contact with

animal-borne illnesses that were previously isolated from most of the population.

4. The increasing number of people with impaired or unhealthy immune systems—caused either by a virus or by certain medical treatments such as organ transplants, chemotherapy, and, possibly, childhood immunizations—which has expanded the fertile breeding ground for these new and frightening threats to our well-being and even our lives.

In a recent newspaper article by medical writer, Phillip E. Canuto, published in *The Beacon Journal* in Akron, Ohio, there is a chilling account of the surge in diseases that defy modern medicine.

One quote in the story from Dr. William Gardner, chairman of the Department of Medicine at Akron General Medical Center, is particularly disturbing:

"When you talk about emerging pathogens, you're just not talking about new bugs," he said, "but new syndromes caused by old bugs." This is evidenced by the surge in pertussis (whooping cough) last year in Cincinnati, as well as a warning from public health officials that a growing raccoon population in the northeastern United States could hasten the spread of rabies. Some might suggest that a horde of locust is the next plague.

Lest we think all of this is not a serious matter, not only in this country but worldwide, we should note that in June 1994, the U.S. Centers for Disease Control and Prevention issued a master plan outlining steps that should be taken to strengthen the ability to identify and fight new infectious threats.

The battle plan lays out a long list of suggestions, from the creation of sentinels to act as a distant early warning of a new disease, to beefed-up laboratories designed to forecast, as well as research, all symptoms of these attackers. Yet a common strategy the medical profession has used against illness is the prophylactic prescribing of antibiotics for hospitalized patients, which means they don't give them antibiotics because of sickness, but in the hopes of preventing illness. Is this a solution? Of course not. Hospitals have become breeding grounds for many antibiotic-resistant bacteria. Staph bacteria are the number one cause of the 2 million infections acquired in hospitals each year. I'm all for the right kind of prevention of illness, but this isn't even close.

Unless this country considers *all* forms of health care and *preventive* methods including chiropractic, improved nutrition, healthier, chemical-free food, and a complete preventative medicine type of health plan, we will be lowered to the ground in larger numbers. The old saying, "What you don't know won't hurt you," couldn't be more false when we're talking about our health-care system.

It seems that not much is being done about this, but, fortunately, there are a few voices crying in the wilderness. A former researcher for the National Institute of Health (NIH), Dr. Jaffee, M.D., Ph.D., pointed out to the director that there were approximately 125 divisions of the organization earnestly researching diseases—but *not one* was researching the study of health. University of Illinois Professor, Marc Happe, Ph.D., also submits that "no antibiotic can be said to have proven successful in truly eradicating any infectious disease in modern times."

What emerges from this controversy is the simple fact that the average person is thoroughly confused about what to do about any of it. As a result, they don't do anything, suffering the consequences of poor health, including premature death.

## THE CHIROPRACTIC APPROACH
## TO THE IMMUNE SYSTEM

Why do so many of our patients with so many different health problems benefit from chiropractic care? It's true that we don't give medicines or perform surgery—so how is the healing possible?

I believe we all understand by now that we have within us a natural healing ability. It is there all the time, sick or well. Chiropractors know how powerful it can be and recognize its importance. The medical journals are filled with stories of people recovering from "incurable" diseases, of spontaneous remissions, and of recoveries that can't be explained.

Do we know why we get sick in the first place? It would seem that if we have this innate ability to heal ourselves, there is no reason why we should suffer the indignities of being sick at all. While it is true that we all possess this incredible healing ability from within, it also appears that there are many factors that can affect it adversely. The primary duty of a doctor, chiropractic or medical, is to raise the patient's natural or innate healing ability so that it can achieve what it was designed to do—naturally heal. One of the most sensible (and effective) alternatives to medication is something I know about firsthand—chiropractic care. Our chiropractic health-care system teaches us that true health does not come from a pill bottle, a lotion, a potion, or any other chemical concoction. True health comes from within. Good health is an indication that the body is functioning properly. We, as chiropractors, correct a very common condition that interferes with the body's proper functions, which causes it to weaken and become susceptible to disease. That condition is called a vertebral subluxation, which you learned about in Chapter 2.

## Improving the Function of Your Immune System

There are many things you can do to bolster your immune system. In many cases, you can even surpass your inherited level of immunity. Fortunately, your immune system acquires new antibodies throughout life. The immune system develops antibodies using its own resources. All it takes to improve the system is a little work and sincere desire. You will not be surprised by now, when I tell you that the best and fastest way to do this is through chiropractic care, exercise, and proper nutrition. There are also other ways to help yourself, such as vitamins, a better mental attitude, herbal therapy, a less stressful lifestyle, and the limited use of antibiotics. The World Health Organization tells us that "the best vaccine against common infectious diseases is an adequate diet," and with this, I heartily agree.

There is mounting substantiation that vitamin and mineral deficiency can lead to decreased immunity and increased infection susceptibility. By now we should all be aware that vitamin and mineral supplementation can boost immunity and build resistance to infection. Our soil is deficient in trace minerals, our food is full of chemicals, and our air is dirty. I doubt I will get many arguments from that statement. For these reasons, I believe we should help our immune systems operate better by taking vitamin and mineral supplements.

Now, let's talk a little about exercise. Oh no, I can hear the groans now. You're asking if you have to watch all those TV exercise shows, buy a Denise Austin exercise tape, and walk five miles every day. Do you have to sweat with the oldies with Richard Simmons? What kind of exercises should you do? How much? What kind is best? How long?

All these questions emerge again and again, along with personal examples of people who have never taken care of themselves, yet are as healthy as horses, and people who have always been "health nuts," but are now dying of cancer. Do any of these sound familiar?

"My grandpa lived to be 94 years old and smoked every day of his life from the time he was 9 years old." *(Of course, he suffered with emphysema for the thirty years before he died, and he couldn't walk across the room without coughing or using his oxygen machine, but he was alive . . . sort of.)*

"My mother ate fatty meat and all those southern lard dishes all her life, and she lived to be 87." *(Well, sure she had high blood pressure, hardening of the arteries, and diabetes. She was in terrible pain much of the time, and suffered something awful before she passed away, but she was . . . living.)*

"The only exercise my grandfather, who lived to be 101, ever got was chasing my grandmother around the house." *(OK, so this one works . . . even though your grandmother may have had to explain to your grandfather why he was chasing her.)*

"My uncle Joe drank whiskey like it was water and lived to the ripe old age of 89." *(The old dude was married five times, never worked at a job longer than six months, was a mean old codger, you couldn't count on him for nothin', nobody liked him, and he was all twisted up with arthritis and had a horrible liver disease when, to everybody's relief, he finally died.)*

We've all known people who have blatantly abused their health for most of their lives and are still walking, or stumbling, around. The rest of the story is that while many of them did live longer without seeming to take care of themselves, they had little quality to the extra quantity of life they lived. Wouldn't it have been much better to have lived that long life and felt *good* at the same time? You know it would! Read more about maintaining your good health in Chapters 10 and 11.

## The Human Drug Store

The human drug store is a great place. I am talking about your very own pharmacy inside your body. Oh sure, I'm kidding, right? No, I'm not kidding. This little drug store makes every medicine you will ever need—antibiotics; painkillers; insulin; natural chemicals to alter your blood pressure and heartbeat; hormones to regulate your digestion, moods, and blood chemistry; and hundreds of other drugs still undiscovered by science. You have them all, and if your system is in the right order, the "drugs" will be dispensed to your system in the proper amount at the proper time without a prescription. And the price is certainly right.

When chiropractors correct vertebral subluxations, we help you to activate your natural, internal healing process without side effects, adverse reactions, or drug dependency. Reduction of spinal nerve stress permits the body to work more naturally and the nerves to function more efficiently.

Most people have never had their spines checked and their subluxations fixed—and possibly never will. This is extremely unfortunate because spinal subluxation has become an epidemic in our society. It is impossible to have 100-percent healing ability when you have spinal nerve pressure. You cannot live up to your highest potential if spinal nerve stress is present. Having a chiropractic checkup, the same way you have a medical or dental checkup, could make the difference between a lifetime of sickness, suffering, disease, and pain, and one of good health, vitality, and strength.

"You mean, if I go to a chiropractor, I'll never get sick?" you ask. Well, wouldn't it be great if going to a chiropractor kept you from getting sick? It may surprise you to discover that the potential is there. Unfortunately, it is difficult in the society in which we now live, to keep our immune systems strong all the time, even with chiropractic care. If you are under chiropractic care, however, and follow the other immune building techniques, you will be much healthier and live a longer life.

We, in the chiropractic health-care field, believe that we have answers to many of today's health questions. We also believe that the greatest insurance policy one can own is preventative maintenance. Having your spinal column checked periodically for spinal nerve stress is one of the most effective ways of living free from disease and maximizing your innate healing potential. Doctors of chiropractic are able to remove interference from the nervous system and allow the energies of life to flow through the body, providing nourishment, strength, flexibility, and balance to allow your own body to do what it was created to do, which is to take care of *you*.

We also know that the other factors that we have discussed in this chapter—good nutrition, vitamin supplementation, and exercise—have to be taken into consideration when striving for a lifetime of good health. And isn't that what we're all doing—striving for a lifetime of good health? How many times do you hear people use the phrase, "as long as I've got good health, nothing else much matters." We also know that if we don't have good health, all the money and all the success does not amount to anything.

The well-worn saying, "Today is the first day of the rest of your life" can take on an entirely new meaning when you face each day in excellent health, free from pain and debilitating disease.

Impossible? Only if you believe it is.

# Chapter 6

# Your Own
# Information Superhighway

*A man finding himself unsure of his location stopped to ask an old farmer how far it was to the nearest town.*
*"Don't know," was the reply.*
*"Well then, what road do I take to get to the nearest town?" the man asked.*
*"Don't know," was again the reply.*
*"Can you at least tell me the name of the town?" the exasperated man asked, with much irritation.*
*"Don't know," came the answer.*
*"You must be terribly ignorant," the stranger said, shaking his head in disgust. "You just don't seem to know anything."*
*"Well, mister," the old farmer said in a low voice. "I ain't lost."*

Our bodies are very much like the complicated super-highway information systems we hear so much about today. Sometimes we don't receive the messages we ask for or receive the ones sent. It may be because of a misunderstanding, a miscommunication, trouble on the lines, or perhaps a case of apathy or ignorance *(don't know—don't care)*. However, the message will get through if the lines are open and the way unobstructed.

To some, this chapter may seem a bit too technical, although I've tried to keep it as simple as possible in order to communicate my thoughts to you as clearly as I can. Chapter 4 discussed the way each part of the body is connected to the other. In this chapter, I will discuss the nervous system and the importance of chiropractic care in regard to this information superhighway inside your body. Most people already believe chiropractic can help bad backs and other related symptoms (see Chapter 4). In this chapter I will explain why and how chiropractic goes that extra mile to help the body deal with many other things that can (and often do) go wrong.

By now, you know that the basis of chiropractic is that the body can and does heal itself. The *actual cause* of your health problems could (and most likely does) come from a problem in your spine since the nervous system (which runs through the spine) controls all the other systems in the body.

## THE NERVOUS SYSTEM

Our bodies are remarkable structures. All of their complex biochemical reactions, all of the activities of over 100 trillion cells, and dozens of interdependent organs are all under the control and care of our amazing nervous system. The central nervous system—brain, spinal cord, and nerves—controls the entire body. The central nervous system is, we might say, *boss.* Certainly it is *in charge.* It is responsible for the way our machines work. Nothing occurs in the body without being cleared by the nervous system.

Energy is created in the brain and directed down the spinal cord in the form of electrical impulses. That is the highway by which messages travel—our own little on-line message center. There are many exits at various points along the spine. The impulses leave the spine between the vertebrae to travel along different nerve paths to organs and tissues to relay whatever communication necessary to operate this magnificent machine.

This is not a one-way street. There is a return cycle, and each part of the body is continually sending messages regarding what is happening at that particular post back to the brain center where it is processed instantly and the answer returned.

If you back into a hot stove, you do not have to wait five or ten minutes while your back-end fries for this information to be sent to the brain, and then have the brain return a message to move away from the stove. Unless there is something terribly wrong with your system, the message is instantaneous—fortunately.

"Move, you fool, you're against a hot stove!"

This is the brain's way of protecting the body, and for the most part it does an excellent job of communication. The brain is an amazing and quite complicated maze. It is part of the most advanced communications system in the universe. IBM, Apple, and Macintosh are all amateurs compared to our nervous systems. The nervous system alone is made up of billions of nerve "wires" that transmit information from the control center to the outermost regions of our body. The brain takes in billions of pieces of information daily about how the body is working and what is going on all around you and processes it according to your needs. It tells the heart how fast to beat. It balances the blood chemistry. It tells you how to throw a Frisbee, how to run after the dog, or how to bite down on a piece of fudge. It reminds you to put on your sweater when you are chilly (even when your mother is not around) and to turn on the air conditioner when you are hot. It tells your eyes to blink, your feet to walk, and your body to fold into a seated position when you see a chair. It stores trillions of memories and is capable of causing you to express the gamut of human emotions, feelings, moods, or creative inspirations. It can cause you to sing, to laugh, to cry, to dance, to run, to get angry, and to smile.

It is claimed that our nerve network is so extensive that if we were to disappear, and only our nerves remained, we would still be perfectly recognizable. We might look like a faded old photograph, but we would bear a remarkable resemblance to the image in our mirror.

*Amazing,* isn't it?

## The Nerves

There are thirty-one pairs of nerves that branch from the spinal column—each one made of millions of fibers less than one-hundredth the size of a human hair. Each one of the nerve trunks passes through an opening called the *intervertebral foramen,* which is located between the vertebrae. It is at this critical juncture that a misalignment, or what your chiropractor calls a subluxation, can cause health problems by impinging on one of these nerve trunks, causing an interference in the highway to the brain. In short, there's a broken wire and the message cannot get through.

In addition to the spinal nerves, our bodies contain twelve pairs of cranial nerves. These nerves include both sensory and motor nerves that radiate to the eyes, ears, face, mouth, jaw, and nose. The cranial nerves also include the vagus nerve, which passes through the neck and chest to the upper part of the abdomen. The cranial nerves work independently from spinal nerves, but they are affected by alterations in the blood supply and receive transmission from bundles of relay stations known as *ganglia* that are directly connected to the spinal nerves.

What this means to you and me is that health problems relating to the ear, eye, and nasal passages—and the head in general—also respond favorably to chiropractic adjustments. This is why that first "official" chiropractic adjustment made by Dr. D. D. Palmer on a deaf patient one hundred years ago restored the patient's hearing.

Some nerves are *sensory nerves*. Sensory nerves carry impulses from our sense organs to our brains. Without them, we would not be able to see; touch; hear; smell; taste; or feel cold, hot, pain, pleasure or any other stimuli. We would be totally cut off from existence as we know it. Other nerves are *motor nerves*. Motor nerves carry impulses from the central nervous system to both voluntary and involuntary muscles, causing them to contract. They also carry impulses to the glands, effecting secretion. If we had no motor nerves, we would be completely paralyzed. Our muscles would not be able to move and our bodies would not respond to any of our commands. We would be vegetables or prisoners in our own bodies. This is why spinal cord damage is so dangerous. The spinal cord does not have the ability to regenerate itself like the peripheral nerves do. So if you sever the spinal cord or have a stroke that essentially kills the part of the brain connected to the spinal cord, you will be permanently disabled. Some nerves are *mixed nerves*, which means that they have both sensory and motor capacities.

Our nerves also regulate our internal automatic processes, such as respiration, sweating, shivering, excretion, internal organ function, digestion, heartbeat, blood supply to the organs, blood pressure control, and every other absolutely necessary function of our bodies.

The more I think about the way the body is made, the more I wonder how anyone can doubt the existence of a Supreme Being. It is amazing and wonderful to realize how wonderfully made we are, and how we are designed to function so well.

Years ago, when Dr. D. D. Palmer said that the normally functioning brain, operating through a sound nervous system, regulates and integrates every body activity down to the workings of the smallest cell; he was ridiculed by members of the medical profession. His theory, on which chiropractic is based, is now not only universally accepted by the scientific community, but is taught in every medical school in the country as well.

## How the Nervous System Works

We know some things about how the nervous system works. Nobody knows everything about how this wonderful system functions, but we have learned many things. We understand general patterns and know that the signals, or impulses, that travel through this superhighway system resemble an electric current that brings power and lights into our homes. We're not sure how this same system is able to store and recall information and think abstractly or creatively, but most of the time it is enough to know that it *does* work!

The nervous system has two main divisions—the *central nervous system* (CNS) and the *peripheral nervous system* (PNS). The central nervous system can be thought of as the command center. It is composed of the brain and the spinal cord. The peripheral nervous system provides the central nervous system with information about stimuli, and the central nervous system coordinates what actions should be carried out. Neither the central nor the peripheral nervous system could function without the other.

The peripheral nervous system is made up of the cranial and spinal nerves (both sensory and motor) that run between the central nervous system and the rest of the body. It is divided into two different systems, the *somatic* and the *autonomic* systems. The nerves in the somatic nervous system transmit impulses, mainly from external stimuli, to the central nervous system and impulses from the central nervous system to all of the skeletal muscles of the body. It is responsible for our voluntary responses. The somatic nervous system is largely responsible for helping the body to adapt to its external environment through its ability to sense what is going on and its motor responses to the external stimuli.

The autonomic nervous system is responsible for detecting internal stimuli and, with the help of the central nervous system, bringing about the appropriate changes. It is responsible for such involuntary actions as cell repair, waste elimination, and digestion. The autonomic system can be further subdivided into two more systems—the *sympathetic nervous system* and the *parasympathetic nervous system*. These two systems work together, or rather against each other, to regulate *homeostasis*, or a balance of functions in the body.

The sympathetic nervous system does such things as speed up the heart and slow down digestion. For example, if a vicious dog begins to chase you down the street, the sympathetic nervous system kicks in, and your heart pounds, your adrenaline increases, and even your hair follicles may stand on end. When the owner comes out and commands the dog to stop (and the dog does), the other set of nerves, which is the parasympathetic nervous system, takes hold and calms you down, slows down the heart, and again speeds up digestion.

*"OK, folks, back to normal."*

The same thing happens if you are on a roller coaster or watching a Steven King thriller. The brain, as smart as it is, can't really tell the difference in real or imaginary threats, so just to make sure, it puts out the signals in any situation.

*"Watch out . . . it's gonna get you!"*

*"Relax, the danger is over."*

Put a little simpler, these two systems produce the *fight or flight* responses, and it is not good to have either one of these out of balance.

If your sympathetic nervous system becomes too dominant, you will be overreactive, nervous, and stressed. If this is not relieved, disease may follow. Of course, if the parasympathetic nervous system becomes too dominant, you may become a little too laid back, or just plain old lazy. Nothing bothers you enough.

Both of these parts of the nervous system reach every tissue of the body. When healthy, they operate with utmost precision, keeping the body's functions in perfect balance. They are especially important in regulating the thymus gland and the spleen, which are known to play an important role in the body's overall immune system. These two organs manufacture lymphocytes (the white blood cells that protect us from viruses and harmful bacteria).

In addition, both of these systems are interconnected through the spinal nerves. Any obstruction or predisposing condition in either system can alter the normal function of the other.

Because of the multiple duties it performs, we know how important the nervous system is. Whether you are gazing at a beautiful sunset, looking both ways before crossing the street, signing your name to a credit card slip, or secreting intestinal fluids to digest the sandwich you enjoyed for lunch; the nervous system is on the job, performing its tasks with speed and precision. Any interference of the transmission of these signals will interfere with the normal function of the body parts as well. A malfunction of the central nervous system will lead to ill health. Understanding how to correct nerve interference and restore the proper energy transmission to the entire body is what chiropractic care is all about.

If there is a breakdown in communication in your nervous system, you do, indeed, have a serious problem. There is a power outage, a tree across the road, static on the line, a broken cog, a missing spark plug, a short circuit. All malfunctions connect to other functions sometimes causing a chain reaction and serious problems in various parts of the body.

The sympathetic nervous system alone influences enzyme activity in the body, the regulation of DNA and RNA, the functions of the glands, circulation, and basic growth and development and the activity of bone cells. Imagine what could happen in the body if anything goes wrong in the sympathetic nervous system. Medical science has documented that depression, rage, fear, and emotional shock can produce a variety of pathological conditions including decreased immune system function, heart problems, stroke, and ulcers.

The brain contains billions of *neurons*, or nerve cells, that transmit information from one part of the nervous system to another. It is mind-boggling (and brain-straining) to try to conceptualize the vast possibilities of this mass inside our heads. It has been said that if all the connecting lines of the huge telephone networks, (AT&T, Sprint, MCI—all those) carrying *all* the conversations, on *every* phone in the world were compared with one brain's "thought communications" system, the networks that comprise the telephone systems would look extremely puny.

Whew! You could hear a pin drop in the fiber-optic community.

## THE BONES THAT HOUSE THE COMPONENTS OF THE NERVOUS SYSTEM

The brain, the spinal cord, and the spinal nerves are all extremely delicate structures, and as such, need the protection of the body's bony framework. The brain is stored in a very safe place inside the head, completely encapsulated by bone for its protection. It is from this vantage point that the brain controls the body and runs the show.

Just as the skull provides a strong protective armor for the brain, the spinal column is the home of the spinal cord, providing a protective bony housing as well. The spinal cord is surrounded by thirty-three rings of bone (*vertebrae*). These bones are stacked up on top of each other much the way a pile of donuts could be stacked. I hope this imagery is quite clear to you without making you too hungry. These bones are all (or should be) stacked in a straight line, providing the canal or highway through which the spinal cord, as well as all the messages it carries, travel. Not only does the spine protect the spinal cord, but it is essentially the skeletal framework that keeps our body upright—much like the framework of a building.

The ancient Greeks thought that people's backs looked like a lot of bumps resembling thorns, which is why they called them *spina*, which is Greek for the word "thorn." The word vertebrae is from the Latin, *vertere*, which means "to turn."

I don't know how many of you are fans of the cartoon *The Far Side*, but there is one particularly humorous panel showing a sign over a fence that reads: "Boneless Chicken Ranch." Behind the fence there are acres of "things" that appear to be blobs of chickens without bones. Without our bones, especially our spines, we'd simply be "blobs" of mass. Think about it. It's not as funny, however, as it is with the chickens.

All of our body mechanics depend heavily upon spinal flexibility with complete harmonious movement of all the components of the spine. The spinal column is divided into sections: cervical (neck), thoracic (mid-back), and lumbar (lower back), plus the sacrum (located between the lumbar and the coccyx) and the coccyx (the tailbone). All mammals have seven neck bones also referred to as cervical vertebrae. Doesn't it seem odd that the tiny guinea pig, the long-necked giraffe, and the human being all have the same number of cervical vertebrae?

The first and second cervical vertebrae are important for the support and motion of the head. The first cervical vertebra, the atlas, which is directly below the skull, supports your head and allows the nodding motion of the head. The second cervical vertebra is called the axis because it permits the turning and tilting of the head.

Summing up, the spinal column, or backbone, is made up of seven cervical (neck) vertebrae, twelve thoracic (mid-back) vertebrae, five lumbar (low back) vertebrae, one sacrum (made up of five fused vertebrae), and one coccyx (made up of four fused vertebrae), giving us twenty-four moveable vertebrae and nine fused vertebrae, for a grand total of thirty-three vertebral segments.

The vertebrae are separated from each other by cartilage cushions called *discs*, which are elastic. They have about the same pliability as your ear lobes do. Reach up and feel them. Much like a shock absorber in your automobile they provide the shock absorption and flexibility of your spine. They also maintain the spaces between the vertebrae, which is necessary for the undisturbed paths of the spinal nerves between the bones.

*Ligaments*, which have been compared to heavy-duty rubber bands, attach the spinal bones together and cover a major portion of each surface (front, rear, sides) of each of the vertebrae. These ligaments are strong enough to maintain the spine and hold it together, while being flexible enough to allow full range of movement.

## CHIROPRACTIC AND THE NERVOUS SYSTEM

Chiropractic frees the nervous system of interference. It gets that tree off the road or that static off the line and opens up the highway for clear passage of the messages to and from the brain, allowing the body to function again as it was meant to do.

When the nervous system is free of interference, it only stands to reason that good health is likely to follow. According to Dr. A. J. Cunningham in the text *Biological Mediators of Behavior and Disease*, "disregulation of the central nervous system is increasingly being implicated as a contributing factor in disease and can adversely affect the hormonal system, the immune system and our general health."

Long before the time of Hippocrates, a healthy spine was recognized as essential to good health. And since the spine is forever married to the nervous system, there is no way to separate the two when it comes to proper health care.

Chiropractic care is the *only* science specifically concerned with the proper care of the spine, the relationship between it and the nervous system, and our overall good health. The spinal column is the main shaft of the body. It is so beautifully designed that the intervertebral foramina between the bones are exactly the correct shape and size to accommodate the big nerve trunks, along with the veins and arteries that pass through them. You don't have to be a nuclear scientist to understand the simplicity of the fact that if the openings are properly maintained, nerve energy from the brain will flow unimpeded through the nerve trunks and onward to eventually reach every cell in the body. If one or more of the vertebrae are out of alignment, the opening becomes smaller as a result of a hard bone impinging on a soft nerve—subluxation—or an obstruction blocking the body's natural functions.

"Help, the passage is blocked, I can't get through!"

What happens if the body is not able to protect and heal itself? Right—you get sick. If the problem is left uncorrected, what do you think happens? You get sicker. If you go to a medical doctor, what happens? You get medicine. And in most cases, what does the medicine do? It covers, masks, or hides the symptoms. It does not work on the cause of the symp-

---

# Did You Know...

... that adverse health effects from inappropriate use of pre-scription drugs add approximately *$20 billion* to the nation's hospital bills?

---

toms—the blocked nerve—but treats the symptoms only. Then, because the pain is no longer there, we think we are cured. Our bodies know better, however. They tried to tell us, but we wouldn't listen. They are hearty, though, and will keep trying. Sometimes the medicine makes us ill, and we simply trade one ailment for another. Listen to the voice of your body. Your innate intelligence is trying to tell you something important.

Listen. *Listen closely.*

An example of the intricate pattern of the body and how it tries to alert you of a subluxation would be if an impinged nerve in your mid-back caused localized pain or weakness in an organ that that nerve serves, such as the colon. This could bring about constipation, diarrhea, spasticity, or colitis, either immediately or, perhaps, later. Chiropractors have discovered that impairment of the proper flow of energy through a nerve is usually followed by a malfunction in the organ that it serves, which causes symptoms.

Recent studies have also shown that the size of a subluxation is not really the issue. It may be large enough to be recognized even by the most untrained eye, or so small that it escapes the attention of all but the most experienced specialist. The degree of displacement has no direct correlation with the amount of nerve interference. If a tiny misalignment inhibits the vital flow of cerebrospinal fluid for impulse transmission, your brain will not get the message. This is why most chiropractors are just as serious about the smaller subluxations as they are about those that would be considered major problems. The resultant pressure on, and possible irritation of, the delicate spinal nerves may increase or decrease the flow of nerve energy to the organs or tissues served by the particular nerve. One of the most dangerous things about the small subluxation is the fact that it may go undetected and uncorrected for years, producing long-term effects that may result in permanent damages to nerves, muscles, organs, or to the spine itself, causing degeneration of the spine.

Unfortunately, many medical doctors overlook (or are unaware of) the subtlety of subluxations. Worse yet, some claim that they are simply figments of the chiropractic community's imagination. This shows a great deal of ignorance and/or arrogance. As far back as 1909, the existence of subluxations and their powerful effects on a patient's health has been documented in medical journals.

For example, the distinguished surgeon James P. Warbasse wrote, "Subluxations of the vertebrae occur in all parts of the spine and in all degrees. When the dislocation is so slight as not to affect the spinal cord, it will still produce disturbances in the spinal nerves, passing off through the spinal foramina."

One of the most exciting areas of study in physical medicine today is what is known scientifically as the *chiropractic subluxation complex* or CSC. Dr. Robert Dishman, D.C., writing in the *Journal of Manipulative and Physiological Therapeutics*, stated, "The 'chiropractic subluxation complex' may now be defined and described as a definite clinical entity having broad and deep implications concerning pathogenesis."

We need a lot more research concerning this complicated system, but, unfortunately, the chiropractic schools do not receive the millions of research dollars annually that medical schools do. Whether this is due to ignorance or is simply another means of control is another story entirely.

I believe we can all understand the spine and nervous system. If I didn't think that, I wouldn't be writing this book. Granted, the relationship between the spine and the nervous system is extremely complex. But in the past few years, people have become increasingly educated about their own bodies and quite willing to put forth that extra effort to find out all they can about good health for themselves and their families. No longer do they simply take the word of their family doctor, or anyone else for that matter, as absolute fact. There is too much at stake. More and more people are beginning to realize that for years they've been lied to or misinformed about their health. No longer can a medical doctor sit back on what he considers his laurels and expect his patients to accept his word at face value. The public is becoming more and more aware of alternative treatments. It is no longer uncommon that the "second opinion" comes not from another medical doctor but from a chiropractor.

Chiropractic has reached the stage where many more people are open to its teachings and practices. It has proven itself to be a painkiller (as opposed to pills), an alternative to surgery, a lifesaver, and an all-around health-care program. It appeals to those who take the time to study its benefits and to reason that if the Creator made their bodies to operate in such an amazing pattern, those functions should be allowed to take their own natural courses.

If someone tells you that you have a lot of nerve, they may mean you have a lot of courage or, perhaps, a lot of irritating qualities. However, our nerves are really an extension of our brain, the center of our being. If we had no nerves, we could not survive. I cannot stress enough how important it is to keep our nervous systems healthy. Without healthy nerves the body is weakened and unable to adapt to environmental and psychological stresses.

So if someone tells you that you've got "some nerve," just smile, thank them, and make sure that all of them are healthy and able to operate without interference.

Keep that information superhighway open!

# Chapter 7

# The "C" Monster

The little boy came running inside the house. He was out of breath and obviously in much distress.

"There's a big horrible monster in the back yard," he finally managed to tell his mother.

The mother, who was quite accustomed to her son's tall tales, looked out the window. There on the lawn was a large shaggy dog, wagging his friendly tail.

"It's just the neighbor's new dog," she said, scolding him for yet another exaggeration. "I'll tell you what. Because you've gotten into the habit of telling untruths, I believe it might be a good idea if you went to your room and prayed to God to forgive you for telling another lie." She also admonished him not to come out until he was forgiven.

The boy did as he was told, but a short time later emerged from his room.

"What are you doing out of your room?" the mother asked.

"I did what you said," the boy answered.

"And did God forgive you for saying the neighbor's dog was a big monster?" she asked.

"Oh yeah," the boy quickly replied. "God said the first couple of times he saw that dog, He thought it was a big old monster, too!"

A re we seeing monsters, too? Sometimes it does seem that they are everywhere, and we often find ourselves looking over our shoulders in fear of what we know to be a threat to us and to those we love. Are there really monsters out there?

Take a walk people!

Am I talking exercise here? No, I'm telling you to take a walk into the various hospitals, medical clinics, and retirement homes in America today. Then think about what you've seen. It won't be a pretty picture. It becomes even more frightening when that walk is down the halls of a children's hospital, where bed after bed is occupied by the light of someone's life—a sick and sometimes dying child. Americans are suffering from all kinds of diseases today, but the number one killer is the dreaded monster we call *cancer*, or the "C" Monster. Unlike the "shaggy dog monster" seen by the little boy, this one is very real, and it is out to devour any one of us.

When we discussed the superinformation highway—our nervous system—and how important it is to our overall good health in Chapter 6, I mentioned that there are many diseases that are caused by that obstruction that keeps the body from doing its job 100 percent. And if it doesn't do its job 100 percent, an illness can occur. Sometimes that illness is cancer.

To see all the pain and suffering of all kinds in our hospitals and rest homes today not only makes me unbearably sad but often physically ill as well. The image of a baby hooked up to all those monitors and tubes and machines is one of the most painful experiences ever to take place in a parent's or a grandparent's life. I'm not saying that some of these methods aren't necessary—lifesavers even—for the child, but you must ask yourself the following questions:

- Could this have been prevented?

- Do we have to get sick like this?

- What actually caused this?

- Is the cure worse than the illness?

- Does our Creator want us sick?

- Has this child ever had an adjustment?

- Has this child ever been checked for a misaligned vertebra?
- Has this child ever had a spinal checkup?
- Are we missing something?
- Does anyone here understand true health?
- Is there a better way?

There *must* be a better way!

What does all this have to do with the problem? you ask. It could have *everything* to do with it. What you may not know is that if that child or other loved one has a subluxation, that subluxation prevents the natural life flow from the brain through the spine to the smallest peripheral tissue cell. By now, you should be well aware that with a subluxation, a patient can become a target for all kinds of diseases—cancer being one of the most fearsome. Can the patient's immune system fight off this terrorist? Yes, but only if the ammunition is available. We have to recognize the importance of prevention, but most of all we have to know the difference between the neighbor's friendly dog and a real monster. *Cancer*—this is one of the real monsters.

Cancer is a killer. I know it. You know it. God knows it. Medical doctors know it. Chiropractors know it. You would find it difficult to find anyone in the entire world who is not aware of the dangers and the ravaging effects of cancer.

The big question is what do we do about this knowledge? Do we just sit and wait for cancer to strike—hoping in the meantime that our luck will hold out, and we will be able to defend ourselves against its curse? Or *maybe* we will not be a target at all. Is there something we can do to prevent this monster, as well as other dangerous diseases, from attacking us? Can we prevent cancer or, at best, help our bodies to help themselves?

I believe we can.

I believe we can.

I *know* we can.

I am concentrating on cancer in this chapter because it is a highly feared disease. To further add to the horror of this disease, in some cases the medical community uses these fears to control us, to actually force us into doing what it wants us to do. Even the word "cancer" is frightening and certainly threatening to our well-being and often to our lives. When John Wayne gave an interview after learning he had cancer, he referred to his illness only as "The Big C." Some refer to cancer as "The Big C" because they cannot bring themselves to face the reality of its horror. Every one of us has been touched in some way by this dreaded affliction, if not in our own personal health, then in the lives of our friends and relatives. Most of us have lost someone we care about to this dreaded disease.

It is chilling to learn that cancer will affect *one out of three* Americans. The American Cancer Society tells us that in 1989 the number of new cancer cases topped the one million mark, with half of those resulting in death.

## A LOSING BATTLE

Early detection is one of the first lines of defense. This is stressed again and again by the medical profession, and, of course, they are correct—to a point. The sooner cancer is discovered, the better the chances of fighting it—and beating it. Unfortunately, even though the medical profession is finding cancer sooner now, their methods of fighting it are the same old, worn-out techniques, and we continue to suffer and die in growing numbers.

It would appear that we are fighting cancer. In the United States alone we spend almost *one-half trillion dollars* per year to fight diseases. Despite this, cancer and heart disease alone take the lives of 4,000 people *every single day!* Heart disease kills twice as many people as cancer, yet we fear the cancer monster more because it causes so much more suffering. The toll mounts even higher when the agony and suffering of the survivors of the victims is counted. Add all this misery to the millions (both adults and children) who suffer from diabetes; emotional breakdowns; arthritis; and diseases of the digestive tract, kidneys, liver, prostate—all our body parts—and it is beyond the scope of our worst nightmares. Does all this strike you as "winning the health war"? I don't think so.

Figures show that the chances of a patient's complete recovery from the dreaded cancer are, in most cases, not significantly better today than they were forty years ago, yet look how much money we keep sinking into research.

It's been said that if you live five years after having cancer treatment, and there are no signs of the cancer, you could consider yourself cured. Well, our diagnosis methods for cancer have improved, and the advertising for early detection did its job. People are getting checkups more frequently, and, therefore, cancer is being detected earlier. That's good. But what isn't good is that the same rate of five cancer-free years is still being used to establish that cancer patients are cured, and that's misleading. Cancer is being detected earlier these days, which means that the cancer cells are removed sooner—before they have a chance to get a firm grip on the body and spread. This means that the few cancer cells that are left will take longer to spread throughout the body. So when five years pass, and there is no sign of any new cancer, the patient is diagnosed as being cured of his or her cancer, when in reality, the patient may not be cured at all, the cancer just may not have gotten a chance to spread yet.

Some chilling statistics were found in the article "Losing the Cancer War," by S. Epstein, published in *USA Today*. "Since 1950, the overall incidence rates have increased by 40 percent. Cancers of the breast, prostate, and colon have escalated 60 percent; in children 30 percent. Less common cancers have increased more than 100 percent."

There is, of course, no *one* answer to the very important question of why we are losing the war on cancer. Many believe it is because modern medicine directs its attention toward the tumor that is in the body, rather than at the body that developed the tumor.

Another theory, which is extremely difficult for most of us to believe, is that the "cancer establishment" (which includes some medical doctors, many pharmaceutical companies, hospitals, and government agencies) promotes highly toxic and expensive drugs, patented by major pharmaceutical firms, which also have close links to cancer care centers. It is unlikely that they would investigate innovative approaches developed outside their own institutions because it would be something they could not patent, control, or—God forbid—make money on.

That would be too horrific to believe, wouldn't it? Still, we have to think about it. If men would start wars for their own personal gain, and we know that they have, then why is it beyond our realm of imagination to think of what they might do for the *billions of dollars* made each year by the pharmaceutical companies?

## THE MEDICAL APPROACH TO CANCER

As I stated before, medical treatment for cancer is tumor-oriented. The only methods of ridding the patient of the intruder, according to the medical community, is to *cut* it out with surgery, *burn* it out with radiation, or *poison* it with chemotherapy. Cut! Burn! Poison! All of these methods greatly diminish the ability of that individual's immune system to function properly. Chemotherapy has been found to decrease the white blood cell count and cause a general inability to fight infections. We are all well aware that surgery, general anesthesia, blood transfusions, and radiation therapy also depress the immune system. And what do we need to fight cancer? You're right . . . a strong and healthy immune system.

The survival rates for some kinds of cancer actually declined because of the more vigorous application of proven methods like toxic chemotherapy, which sometimes kills those patients on whom it is used. The power of chemotherapy lies in its ability to "kill" the cancer. At the same time it is killing all the other cells around it and weakening the immune system with every chemical treatment. Chemicals placed in the body are toxic, and it is often a toss-up whether the cancer cells will die before the patient succumbs and the immune system will be strong enough to fend off the toxin in the body or not. If a patient has to submit to chemotherapy—and sometimes it is necessary as the last resort—then it is absolutely imperative that that same individual has an immune system second to none, because he or she will need every weapon in his or her health arsenal to win this fight. It literally means the difference between life and death.

Chemotherapy is *one* way to fight cancer. Yet we have to look at the whole picture. A pre-eminent German biostatistician, after an exhaustive review of thousands of cancer research studies, made the following statement: "Faith in chemotherapy is a fixed dogma that cannot be supported by the scientific evidence. Chemotherapy is incapable of extending . . . the lives of patients suffering from the most common organic cancers (breast, intestine, bladder, lung, pancreas)."

I don't think I can repeat too many times that you are the one in charge of your own health. You are the one who will suffer if you do not take care of yourself. You are the one who will suffer the pain of whatever dreaded disease that befalls you. You must begin by maintaining your body and preventing as many illnesses as possible.

I'm often reminded of the story of the two automobiles that came off the assembly line the same day. They were both the same model and style, even the same color. They were sold to two very different people on the same day. The first owner simply adored his new vehicle and cared for it in such a manner that brought envy to the other car, which was purchased by a gentleman who was extremely busy. The first owner washed, waxed, and pampered his car regularly, and he changed the oil as indicated by the manual. He used the best grade of gasoline and tuned up the engine right on schedule.

The second owner gave little thought to his method of transportation. He simply got into the car and drove it when he wanted to go somewhere. He put whatever gas was handy in it and checked the oil when the red warning light came on. When the car wouldn't start or the engine missed, he would take it into the station for a tune-up. As he watched his car being towed off to the junkyard, he complained that "they just don't make cars the way they used to."

Even though we are not machines, and there is really nothing with which we can compare the human body due to its uniqueness, I will compare the way we treat our bodies to the car example. We will usually get the type of health we work toward. It's a matter of taking the time and concentrated effort to *make the difference.* We can take care of ourselves and remain "showroom" new, or we can end up in the junkyard before our time.

Of course, you may not get this type of information from your average medical doctor. They truly believe the body needs help (interference) in order to be healthy. They don't believe very much in the effectiveness of good nutrition, vitamins, or exercises. As a rule, they believe the body is going to break down, and they will have to fix it. I never cease to be amazed at the egotistical attitude of many of our country's extremely intelligent medical doctors. This makes it very difficult to get them to consider another way of health care.

## Medical Breakthroughs

We are being told by the media that there are medical break-throughs every day. We would all like to believe that one day soon, the dreaded "C" monster will be banished from our lives completely. And this is what we're supposed to believe. This is why we willingly donate millions and millions of dollars, as well as our time, energy, and efforts every year for research to wipe out this dreaded disease. And if we could succeed, it would be worth every penny—and much more. But that's not what's happening. We know that is not happening. We *hear* that it is, but we *know* better. Unfortunately, if we continue to put strong, powerful, and deadly drugs inside our bodies, then we also run the risk of killing ourselves as well. What we have to understand is that the "cure" comes from inside—and those so-called spontaneous remissions are simply the body's way of taking care of itself.

So, are we near a cure for cancer—medically speaking? Given the past records, I'm afraid this will not happen through medical research. While it is true that in laboratories across the country, diligent and dedicated people work unlimited hours in search of that effective vaccine, that perfect medicine, or that powerful magic bullet that will be able to drop the dreaded monster in its tracks; we can only shake our heads sadly and report that they have not yet found it.

The monster keeps coming. Why? I believe that it is because the researchers are looking in the wrong places. Again, you cannot work *outside the body, in,* but you must work *inside the body, out.* This is the foundation upon which D. D. Palmer, and later, his son B. J. Palmer, built chiropractic health.

Now and then we see a headline that causes us to have hope that there will be a cure, but statistics prove to us that most of the time these hopes turn out to be false. That  false hope that a cancer cure is near is still held out to us. We are being

# *Did You Know...*

. . . that what chiropractors have been saying for years and years is now being touted as "big news"? In the May 29, 1997 issue of *USA Today,* the cover story states that according to a new analysis just out, despite twenty-six years of work and $30 billion spent, the American government's so-called "War on Cancer" has been lost—it has failed to substantially reduce death rates from the disease.

The next big news flash in the same story is that researchers have come to the conclusion that the battle should shift to another front: *prevention.* Is anyone listening?

According to the results of a study just released and reported in the latest issue of the *New England Journal of Medicine,* John Bailar and Heather Gornick of the University of Chicago contend that their analysis shows that the effect on mortality of new treatments for cancer has been "largely disappointing." They added that "the most promising approach to the control of cancer is a national commitment to prevention, with a rebalancing of the focus and funding of research."

Bailar and Gornick found that the nation's cancer death rate grew by 6 percent between 1970 and 1994—from 189.6 deaths per 100,000 people to 200.9 per 100,000 peaking in 1991, and then declining by 1 percent in 1994. All of the statistics have been adjusted to account for the aging of the population. Researchers disagree, however, over how much the improvement between 1991 and 1994 is due to novel cancer treatments, to the lesser number of smokers, and to early detection of tumors while they are still small.

"I think we have to give very serious thought to alternatives," Bailar concluded.

led by this "hope" into believing that the end of the dreaded cancer is on its way.

Billions of dollars have been spent and years of research have been invested, yet we still have untold suffering and millions of deaths to show for these untiring efforts. When you hear about "progress" being made in cancer research, remember these words as published in the *New England Journal of Medicine*. The article was written by John C. Bailar, editor of the *Journal of the National Cancer Institute* and co-author of a report assessing the overall progress against cancer from 1950 through 1985:

> These data taken alone provide no evidence that some thirty-five years of intense and growing efforts to improve the treatment of cancer have had much overall effect on the most fundamental measure of clinical outcome—death. Indeed, with respect to cancer as a whole, we have slowly lost ground. Incidence of cancer is also increasing, suggesting a failure to prevent or control new or current causes of cancer.

And as if that were not frightening enough, it was stated later in the text that the effort toward improvement in cancer treatment must be judged as a qualified failure. ". . . The reason for this failure needs to be carefully assessed, but in the meanwhile, it may be that our approach to cancer needs to be changed." The study further contends that for future consideration, "the most promising areas are in cancer *prevention*—rather than treatment."

Another renowned medical expert, Dr. John Cairns of Harvard, is also of the opinion that the battle against cancer is being lost. He is quoted as saying: "My criticisms (are) that the cancer treatment and research is giving the public an endless succession of breakthroughs and solutions that aren't really that at all."

This is almost as scary as the monster itself. After a while, we begin to become somewhat paranoid, and we begin to wonder who we can trust *totally*. Is there no one human being out there who does not have his or her own agenda, or is *not* after his or her own personal gain or interests in some way? I think if we have a problem trusting *specific people*, then perhaps we can trust a principle instead: The body was made in a way that it can heal itself (when treated with respect and care) from *every illness upon the face of the earth*. It is my belief that we must understand, strive for, and accept this basic principle of life.

The body heals itself.

When a patient goes into spontaneous remission, many medical doctors will take credit for it. A person who gets well after he or she has been declared terminally ill often doesn't go back to the doctor and is not included amongst those who have managed to overcome this scourge. Those who do return to the doctor with the good news, will sometimes be told that the doctor made a mistake in his or her diagnosis. Spontaneous remissions are often thought of as unexplainable or as flukes—mysteries to medical science. There are far more of these unexplained cures and remissions than previously believed or reported in medical journals. Most of the patients know what happened. They know there was a higher power at work, or they turned to alternative methods of treatment—sometimes doing nothing more than changing their diet, getting plenty of exercise, and changing their lifestyles in such a way that improved their general health and the health of their immune systems, which in turn, went to battle for them. The ability to beat a disease, especially cancer, is often attributed to that patient who has this innate sense of self-preservation and survival traits, who seeks solutions rather than gives up. The survivors seem to be those who interpret problems as re-directions, not as failures. What we also have here is that intangible power of higher intelligence at work.

There are some cures, or some relief from some illnesses. Still, I'm sure you've heard that old saying about the cure being worse than the illness. Cancer is a prime example of that. In many cases the treatment is contrary to the dynamics of the human body. Furthermore, some treatments are attempted simply because medical technicians have to *do something,* or the general public will start to ask questions about where the billions of dollars are going.

It is incomprehensible to most of us that some human beings could do this to other human beings for financial (or any other) gain, but, unfortunately, it happens. This is not to say that there aren't many brilliant and dedicated researchers working long, tedious hours in lonely laboratories, racing against the death clocks to try to discover a real cure for many of our diseases, including cancer. We know this is true. They are most often good and decent people, striving to do good and decent work, but some may well be misguided in their quest to help their fellow human beings.

## THE CHIROPRACTIC APPROACH TO CANCER

I'm not saying there are no answers to the cancer question. I do believe there are alternative choices, and I cannot repeat this too many times—there is *prevention*! We must think of our health care as a preventative measure rather than one of fighting disease. The odds are against us when the disease gets a firm hold on us, but if we remain strong with our immune systems intact, then we reduce our chances of serious illness many times over.

In his book *Chiropractic Alternative*, Nathaniel Altman argues that an interference-free nervous system helps fight cancer. "John C. has cancer, but after four months of chiropractic care, he is in remission. Does that mean that chiropractic cures cancer? A responsible chiropractor would answer this in the negative, but proceed to ask a more important question: Can a physiologically sound organism, freed from dis-ease and nerve interference, fight cancer? The answer to this is yes."

Altman went on to offer an excerpt from an article published in *TIME* magazine that suggested a relationship between the immune system and cancerous growth. They reasoned that, in addition to protecting the body from invaders, the immune system has the duty to police cell growth and prevent the survival and reproduction of abnormal or "outlaw" cells.

Although chiropractors have never made any claims that chiropractic is a cancer therapy, there is a correlation between chiropractic care and the remission of cancer. This theory is shared by medical authority, Robert Mendelsohn, as is evident in his foreword to *Spasm*, by John C. Lowe. "Indeed to this day I am frustrated at the ability of chiropractors to achieve 'spontaneous remission' in patients with heart disease, arthritis, cancer, and other serious ailments. It seems that we M.D.s do not get our fair share. Why must I advise patients: If you want a spontaneous remission, see a chiropractor."

If you've read this far in this book—or if you've only read this chapter— you can use your own common sense and realize that if you have cancer, it is essential that you have a healthy nervous system and a strong immune system. Do we know how to attain a strong immune system? Of course we do. It is achieved by the nervous system through a healthy spinal column that is free of subluxations.

The achievement of a healthy immune system involves a fight that cannot be fought passively or halfway. Your body needs every ounce of positive input to help fight not only the "C" Monsters but all the monsters that beset us. This fight includes changing to a healthy diet, exercising, and adapting a lifestyle that will not sap the energy of your immune system. If you are under medical care, alternative care, or both, you need to be well informed about all the alternatives in the health-care field. Too many studies (and healthy patients) have proven that chiropractic has a "boosting" effect on the immune system. Your body is much more able to maintain its internal environment with less spinal stress.

A study published in a 1991 article in the *New England Journal of Medicine* found no difference between the survival rate of individuals who had medical treatment for cancer, and the rate of those treated with alternative therapies. However, this study was found to be flawed because the alternative care patients had first been subjected to immune system-damaging surgery, chemotherapy, and radiation before being given over to alternative care. We can only imagine how much better they could have done had their immune system been able to start out on equal footing with the cancer.

Again, we have to keep this immune system in tip-top shape. How do we do this? By *taking care of ourselves!* I cannot repeat it too many times. We must treat our bodies as though our lives depended on it—because they do. We must learn and practice good nutrition, we must exercise, and we must keep our bodies as free from chemicals and foreign substances as possible. In addition, we need regular chiropractic care to help keep subluxations away from our spines, allowing our bodies to operate in the way they were created to. This will keep our immune systems strong, healthy, and ever combat-ready. When the body has to fight cancer, it needs every bit of help it can get!

R.W. Moss, in *The Cancer Industry*, wrote, "The continuing failure of orthodox medicine to deal satisfactorily with the major forms of cancer guarantees the growth of nonconventional approaches . . . among them all may well be some methods of great benefit to cancer patients. It is the job of the true scientist . . . to look at all methods and claims. . . . A million new cases a year demand no less."

Regardless of your preconceived ideas and opinions about chiropractic, you owe it to yourself to study the facts—and more importantly, to talk to those who are chiropractic patients with successful results to report.

No responsible chiropractor will promise that they can "cure" cancer. What we do believe is that chiropractic is beneficial to a cancer patient, whether or not he or she is under the care of a medical doctor.

In the *International Review of Chiropractic*, Pennsylvania chiropractor Dr. Ted Koren pointed out that cancer is "the result of a body not working correctly for many years." Removing nerve interference with chiropractic adjustments may help a body to regain its proper working order. If it works properly, it has a better chance of fighting off cancer or various other diseases. Dr. Koren also states that an uninterrupted nerve supply will give the patient greater natural resistance, thereby avoiding iatrogenic disease, which is often a consequence of cancer therapy.

What I am saying here is that if the body is internally strong, it can and does fight off the beginning cancer cells daily. It is when the body is in a weakened state that the cancer cells win out over our own protective cells.

Let's use someone as an example—someone we all knew, respected, and loved—actor Michael Landon, or Little Joe Cartwright, as many of us came to know him. He was diagnosed with cancer some time ago, and shortly thereafter we read of his death in the newspaper.

We have to ask ourselves if the *day before* Michael started having pain or symptoms, was he *healthy* or was he *sick*? Did his cancer manifest itself in one day? Could it be that on Monday there was not a trace of the cancer in his body—no pain, no symptoms—then on Tuesday, there it was? Not likely. His cancer began long before he had pain. Pain was merely a symptom, a sign that something was wrong. Unfortunately, by the time the symptoms manifested themselves, it was too late for Little Joe. Even though he appeared to fight a diligent battle, he lost. How much better it would have been if he could have been aware of all the preventative measures before the dreaded disease got a death grip on his body.

When a patient suffers certain symptoms or pain, what usually happens? It is not uncommon, at first, for the person to simply hope the pain will go away on its own. He or she ignores it, or tries to smother it with over-the-counter aids or prescription medicines until the pain sometimes subsides for a while. When it returns, the patient knocks it out again and again until he or she can no longer do that and then finally has to face the fact that he or she must deal with whatever is causing this problem. The patient will then go for tests in attempts to determine the cause of the pain. Finally, after a tremendous amount of prodding, testing, and probing, the doctor gives the cancer diagnosis. The doctor has found the cause of the pain, the cause of the nausea, the cause of the weight loss, and the cause of the suffering. Terror strikes as the patient hears the dreaded "C" word.

After a time patients accept that verdict, knowing that it often ends with a death sentence. But do they ask themselves, or do we ever ask ourselves what *caused* the cancer? We wonder, of course, and sometimes a patient will ask the doctor why. Often the doctors will say it is environmentally or chemically induced, or perhaps they will sadly admit that they really don't know what caused it. Some go as far as to say that if they knew what caused it, they could better treat it. Unfortunately, they don't know. They also don't know why the cancer grew in the liver and not the stomach; in the bone and not the prostate. Why didn't it attack the kidney? Or the colon? With the exception of lung cancer caused by smoking, there is almost a "who knows?" attitude when it comes to the causes of cancer.

Nerve interference allows the cells to change abnormally. Nerve interference weakens the body so that the bad cells can proliferate. Nerve interference is the fundamental cause of disease.

If you have strong life flow from the brain cell to the nerve cell and the tissue cell, then wherever that life flow goes, that part of your body remains strong. Conversely, if you have strong life flow from the brain cell to the nerve cell, but due to a misaligned vertebra (subluxation) the life flow from the nerve cell to the tissue cell (in the liver, for example) is impeded, interrupted, interfered with, slowed, shut down, stunted, hampered, or repressed; that liver will become weakened because it is not getting the energy it needs to function the way our Creator meant it to. So guess what happens next? Sickness.

Do you believe disease strikes strong organs and tissues or weakened organs and tissues? Disease strikes the area of greatest weakness. You've heard the saying that a chain is only as strong as its weakest link. If you pulled on that chain, where would it break? It would break at the weakest place. That's the way your body works. You will develop sickness or disease in your body in the weakest area—not your stronger areas. The bottom line is if you keep your body's immune system strong, you will be healthier. If you are healthier—then you are *not sick!* I just can't speak much plainer than that.

What it all comes down to is the body healing itself—and in order to do that with a disease as deadly and unyielding as cancer, it needs every one of its fighters in top form, with all the firepower available. It is a war we cannot afford to keep losing!

And, yes, there is a *better* way to ward off the monsters.

# Chapter 8

# ...And the Other Illnesses

*It is not the disease, but neglect of the remedy, which generally destroys life.*

—a Latin saying

Backaches—that's what the chiropractor fixes, right? Right. But, there's a lot more. Although, isn't that enough?

Those who suffer from this most painful condition know that backaches are among the most devastating and debilitating illnesses known to man or woman. I've had a lot of women tell me that the pain of childbirth was nothing compared with the pain they have from what some call "just a plain old backache." Granted, it is a serious and painful condition, but it is far from the only reason a chiropractor has for existing, nor is it the only reason to go to a chiropractor's office.

Even those who are more informed about chiropractic care can sometimes think no further than muscle spasms, whiplash, arthritis, rheumatism, sciatica, gout, headache, postural deformities, sclerosis, tennis elbow, knee pains, sports-related injuries, and various other joint-related problems.

Even if these problems were the *only* conditions chiropractors helped, this would be a great beginning to good health and pain-free living. Most people know chiropractors help these problems, but what about other ailments?

We have discovered that chiropractic care can have a very positive effect on many other illnesses. My good friend, Dr. Rick

Franks in Atlanta, Georgia says, "If everyone knew the benefits chiropractic had to offer, then every office would have a waiting list of people." I couldn't agree more.

Patients do come to us for such diverse conditions as asthma; heart problems; gynecological problems; stomach conditions; and bowel, prostate, kidney, bladder, gallbladder, eye, ear, nose, and throat conditions—all of which can be helped by chiropractic health care. Unfortunately, many people go first to their medical doctors for these problems, so by the time we see them, their problems have worsened. We can still get results, but it takes a lot longer than if the patient had tried the easiest and most sensible route first.

By now, I believe I have firmly established that chiropractic is a viable health-care alternative, designed to help the body's system work the way nature intended it to work. And if it does that, the patient will be able to withstand many of the diseases that plague us today.

All of our major organs are closely linked to the nervous system, which radiates from the spine. A wide variety of visceral disorders that occur when spinal subluxations cause nerve interference can be greatly improved by chiropractic care.

Although space does not permit me to go into each of these disabilities individually, we will try to cover some of the most common ones, beginning with the all-too-frequent and aggravating headache.

## HEADACHES

What do you think is one of the most frequent complaints I hear in my office?

"I have a *terrible* headache."

Headache is our most common pain, and most people get one at least occasionally. Unfortunately for about 20 percent of the population, headaches are more than an occasional discomfort. They are completely debilitating, chronic, and recurrent. There are more than twenty kinds of headaches, and the migraine even has five subvarieties. Studies have shown that there are certain types of personalities that are prone to more headaches than other personalities. Each type of headache has different reasons for its occurrence.

Confusing? Gives you a headache just thinking about it, doesn't it?

Fortunately, I don't get headaches too often. When I do get one, it is usually brought on by stress. An adjustment gets rid of them for me. Sometimes, however, there's not a chiropractor available, or I can't take time away from my patients, and I have to suffer with the pain. That's when I wonder how anyone can put up with headache pain for days, sometimes weeks at a time, without at least giving chiropractic a try.

## Causes of Headaches

There are some who fear that a headache is a pain directly of or from the brain. The fact is, however, that the brain, most of the membranes surrounding it, and even the skull bones, do not feel any pain at all. That is why sometimes during brain surgery the patient is fully awake (with only a local anesthetic to numb the scalp) and talking to the doctors while his or her brain is being cut, probed, and moved about. So, I believe in most cases we can rule out a "sick" brain causing a headache.

When the pain-sensitive structures of the head—the arteries and veins of the brain and the skull, the dura matter (tissues) covering the brain, and the cranial nerves—are infected, inflamed, stretched, pulled, compressed, or irritated; you get a headache. While there may be other reasons for a headache, these are the most common reasons.

Headaches due to inflammation or irritation of cranial nerves can be caused by inhaling the fumes of noxious chemicals, by looking at intense bright lights, or by sinus conditions or eye problems. Some headaches are associated with high blood pressure, food allergies, diseased teeth, ear problems, brain tumors, vision problems, fevers, infections, and/or epileptic seizures. Still others can be brought about by hangovers from the side effects of alcohol or drugs (prescription, nonprescription, or recreational). Another common type of headache is the *posttraumatic stress headache* that may occur after an accident. There is also the common muscle tension or nervous headache normally caused by unusual emotional stress or tension. In addition to all of these, there are headaches caused by invasive medical procedures, surgeries, and testing.

When I was a student in my senior year at Life Chiropractic College, I attended a seminar at a local hotel. Directly across the hall, there was a seminar of some kind for medical doctors. A couple of times during the weekend, breaks for both seminars came at the same time. During one of these breaks, I started talking with one of the medical doctors. He almost immediately asked me if chiropractic could help people with headaches. I told him it could and that headaches were one of the main reasons people sought chiropractic care. Immediately, he began to question how chiropractic could possibly help headaches, since we used no drugs to help with the pain. It was then that I realized that what had started out as a pleasant exchange between two professionals had suddenly turned a corner. He *informed* me in a most unfriendly tone that there were *many* reasons why people had headaches. He named several, such as sinus and vision problems, stress, and high blood pressure, causes *only* medical doctors treat. I knew that, of course, and tried to tell him I did, but due to his condescending attitude, I could tell he assumed that I knew very little about anything except adjusting backs.

"What about tumors that cause headaches?" he asked then, looking me straight in the eye, as though we were in a staring match. It was evident that he thought I would know nothing about tumors or *anything* of a medical nature for that matter, and he was hoping to make me look stupid and uninformed.

"Yes," I told him, "tumors can cause headaches . . . *but* . . . what caused the tumor?"

He stood there for a moment, digesting my question as though it had never occurred to him. Finally, he replied that a lot of things can cause a tumor . . . and tumors can cause headaches. Well, we had already established that.

I agreed with him that a lot of things can cause tumors but pointed out to him that chiropractic works on the idea that the nervous system controls *everything* in the body, and a weakened nervous system would allow disease processes to happen because the weakened body could not fight it off.

He looked at me for a moment, then turned on his heel and walked away without another word. I may not have made a conversion, but I could tell that I had set his thoughts in motion. I believe he was considering things that had not been a part of his training or thought process until our conversation. He didn't really understand the concept of seeking the cause of dis-ease. He was totally into treating *symptoms*. I hope he started looking deeper into sickness, dis-ease, and real health. Maybe he even turned the word *prevention* over in his mind as well.

## The Horrible Migraine

If you have ever had, or know anyone who has had, migraine headaches, you know they are not a minor affliction. This malady occurs in 6 to 8 percent of the population and is best described as the *chronic headache* or the *migraine syndrome*. The word "syndrome" refers to a number of symptoms that go together and often arise before the headache actually hits. These may include dizziness, visual problems (spots before the eyes), redness, swelling, muscle contractions, irritability, tears in the eyes, vomiting, constipation, and/or diarrhea. The duration of time can run from a few minutes to a few days, and the severity can range from minor discomfort to immobilizing pain and extreme agony. The location can vary from the temple, which is the most common location, to anywhere in the head, face, or neck.

Through years of performing adjustments, chiropractors have learned how to cope with this most debilitating affliction. Patients of mine who have gained relief from migraines are easily some of the most grateful people I've ever met.

## The Cluster Headache

Suddenly, you feel an intense, throbbing pain arising high in one nostril and spreading behind the eye on that side of the face. You have what is known as a *cluster* headache. Sometimes your forehead is also affected, and the attacks tend to occur from once to several times daily—in clusters—lasting for weeks, or even months. They may subside as quickly as they came, and you cannot imagine what caused them to come—or to go. You just hope you never encounter them again.

Again, I must stress that a healthy body begins with a healthy spinal column. Even if you are seeing other doctors—

medical or alternative—it is still advisable to try chiropractic. In some people, we find that any kind of headache pain disappears very quickly with chiropractic adjustments; while in others, the pain may not go away immediately. The body has to heal its damaged tissues, and often this takes more time than people want to spend. The alternative, however, is that they may spend a lot of time with that cluster or migraine headache instead.

## Take Two Aspirin . . .

Americans lay hundreds of millions of dollars a year on the counters of drug stores across the country trying to get rid of that pesky old headache. Our most common headaches are usually treated with prescribed and over-the-counter painkillers. Aspirin and other over-the-counter remedies are usually used for low intensity pain, while more powerful compounds, including codeine phosphate, ergotamine tartrate, and methysergide maleate are prescribed for the more severe headaches.

The treatment of a headache should depend on the cause, but we are conditioned to pop a couple of pills and hope it goes away. When it does not, we may pop two or three more.

## Chiropractic and Headaches

In many cases, chiropractic care is a wonderful alternative to pill popping, especially for those who suffer often from chronic and debilitating headaches. Chiropractic is not a drug, a therapy, nor is it even considered a treatment for headaches. Yet a lot of people go to a chiropractor for headaches.

All too often, the standard medical approach to some illnesses is to treat the symptoms without considering the cause. Headaches are a perfect example. I have patients who have been swallowing painkillers for years, and while they often offer temporary relief, the headaches—and the cause—are still there. What's even worse, the medicine may mask underlying and extremely serious problems. The constant use of drugs not only risks dependency but can cause serious side effects and keep the actual cause hidden.

I cannot emphasize strongly enough that pain is almost al-

ways _a warning signal_. When your body sends out a pain sig-
nal, it is trying very hard to tell you something! It is making
its own, sometimes desperate, 911 call to your brain headquar-
ters. It is trying to communicate to you, the only way it can,
that something is wrong inside your body. If you simply tell it
to shut up, or you put it on hold with an aspirin or other
painkiller, you are ignoring the warnings nature meant for you
to heed.

Chiropractors are the only healing professionals who are
specifically trained to analyze and correct spinal nerve stress.
Since spinal nerve stress is now reaching epidemic proportions,
it has been called "a silent killer." At the same time that it is
weakening the body, lowering vitality, and lessening its resistance to disease; it is opening the door for all kinds of invaders
inside our bodies—and the victim doesn't suspect a thing!

"She wasn't even sick . . . she just died."

"He always seemed so healthy . . . worked right up to the
day before he died."

"I can't believe that a person who always seemed to feel so
good is gone."

"There was _never_ anything wrong with him."

Sound familiar?

Well, you can bet these people had symptoms. Chances are
they just ignored them. In chiropractic, the five danger words
are "Maybe it will go away." We have been taught to be tough,
suck it up, and not to be a baby to the point where, all too
often, we wait too long before seeking help for our health problems. How many times have you seen written on a tombstone,
"He was our beloved father who never complained about his
pain"?

When your body speaks to you, whether it is through a
headache or any other simple pain, it is _telling you something important!_ Something is wrong! While it is true we are not going
to go through life completely pain-free, we need to _listen_ to
(and heed) the voice of our inner health-care representatives, or
that amazing innate intelligence that is policing our bodies
every second of every day, searching for intruders out to do us
harm.

The vast majority of people have been to their medical doctors for the same health problems for which they finally seek

chiropractic help. Some figures suggest the number of people who seek chiropractic care after first trying medical care is as high as 90 percent. People give medical doctors numerous chances to help them. They spend hundreds, even thousands, of dollars and take prescription after prescription—many of which are downright dangerous, all of which have side effects. Finally, still hurting, they seek out chiropractic care, usually because someone who cared about them told them how chiropractic helped them. A direct referral is the way in which chiropractic has grown all these years. It is satisfied, pain-free patients telling sick, hurting, suffering people how chiropractic offered them a better way to good health. It is extremely satisfying for me to see my patients who have become great advocates of chiropractic care bring in their friends and relatives because they know how much it can help even the long-term sufferers.

As a result of these long-term problems, chiropractors don't get many "easy" health problems with which to work. We get a lot of sick, suffering patients in extreme pain. With three strikes (or more) against him or her, the chiropractor has to work twice as hard to undo whatever damage may have been done, as well as deal with a problem that has had months, sometimes years, to progress to an advanced stage.

You would think that with odds like that, chiropractic care would get the blame for the patient not being able to get better sooner. Sometimes that happens, but for the most part, the patients begin to see and feel improvements where there had been none before.

It is my hope that someday people will bring their children into a chiropractic clinic to be checked the same way they take them to a medical doctor or the dentist for other checkups, so they can grow up healthy and ready to meet a hectic and stressful world. When this happens, there will be much less likelihood of the large numbers of adults sick and in pain because they have been taking care of themselves from childhood up. Then they would only have to worry about accidents and other trauma care problems, which may have been caused by getting run over by a truck or being carried to the top of the Empire State Building and dropped by a great, big, ugly ape.

The importance of spinal adjustment for headache pain or

various other types of pain is not simply a "theory" shared by the chiropractic industry. Independent researchers have noted the relationship between the spinal column and headaches. A study of 6,000 patients who suffered recurring headaches for two to twenty-five years showed that cervical spine trauma was the most important factor in the cause of headache and should be suspected in every nonspecific type of headache. Another dramatic study of childhood migraine sufferers found spinal care to be especially effective. As far back as 1933, noted pathologist N. T. Ussher found that spinal misalignment could produce pathological changes that caused headaches as well as many other disease conditions.

Researchers have also found the cervical spine (or the neck) to be of particular interest in relation to headaches. In the *Journal of Manipulative and Physiological Therapeutics (1989),* an article entitled "Spinal Manipulation and Headaches of Cervical Origin" by H. T. Vernon stated, "The body of literature supporting a cerviogenic origin of headache is substantial, and the case made for greater recognition of the involvement of the cervical spine is compelling."

In other words, the scientific evidence supports the chiropractic claim that spinal care is essential for those suffering from headaches. Additionally, more and more research into our methods is continuing. Chiropractic spinal care is essential for anyone who suffers from chronic or even somewhat frequent headaches. Chiropractors strive for that healthy spinal column, which is the first line of defense against headaches, as well as a maelstrom of other diseases.

## CHIROPRACTIC AND THE HEART

I have devoted an entire chapter to cancer (Chapter 7) and much of this chapter to headaches. While I repeatedly emphasize that chiropractic is not a treatment as much as it is a preventative means of health care, we find that there are still many who don't understand chiropractic care in general.

Healthy people are usually not concerned with, nor do they brag about, how good they feel. There is not even a word in the English language for those who talk all the time about their lack of ailments and general good health. Hypochondriacs or genuinely unhealthy people do not hesitate to tell you over and over how much *this* bothers them and how much *that* hurts, sometimes to the point of exasperation. We've all heard Aunt Polly tell her stories about her operations until we felt we were becoming ill ourselves. It was, from her accounts, a real adventure—painful though it was. It is at these times that we have to wonder if there are people who really and truly enjoy, or derive some perverse pleasure from, being sick. Granted, an illness of any kind does occupy a large part of our minds most of the time, and we tend to speak of that which is the ruling portion of our lives.

As is the case with all of your organs, your heart has a tremendous ability to heal itself. Certain things have to happen first, however. You've heard it before, and I'll state it again. Most people need to make lifestyle changes. I am absolutely amazed at the number of people who, after a serious heart attack, will eat and drink exactly the way they did before the attack. They still fail to exercise, cannot give up the cigarettes, and continue to rush headlong into the stress and strain that put them flat on their backs in the intensive care unit in the first place.

A lot of times I sit down to talk with new patients in my office who have come to see me with a painful lower back, only to discover that they had just had multiple bypass heart surgery. They will tell me that they are taking all of their medication but have made no other lifestyle changes. I ask patients like this if their medical doctor hadn't suggested some changes. Often they say he or she hasn't, or if they did, they did not insist their suggestions be heeded. Everybody knows that smoking is bad for you, exercise is good, and a good nutritionally sound diet is even better, but as far as stressing these things to a heart patient, it is not done often enough or strongly enough.

I try to explain to these patients that their bodies are talking to them—screaming and yelling at them, in some cases— but they just shrug it off. After all, they've had *surgery*. Isn't that enough? Their bodies are telling them that the next warning may be a fatal heart attack. Heart attack survivors can really consider themselves fortunate—and forewarned. Their bodies told them that whatever they were doing *before* the heart attack *wasn't good enough.* If this happens to you, you need help. You need changes. You need to take this warning seriously and help yourself. It's a sin the way many medical people treat their patients. It is as though they are saying, "Do what you want, then come back to me, I'll fix it." Sometimes things go beyond the realm of "being fixed."

Some will even deny that there needs to be any sort of a change in their lifestyle. We all know what usually happens to them, and we discuss it in sad whispers at the funeral home amid the lovely flowers that all their good friends sent.

There are always some, however, who will make some type of effort to change, usually to appease their spouses or children who desperately want them to live to a happy and healthy old age. I can't help but wonder if they don't realize what a tremendous warning has been dispatched to them with the heart attack. The message is very clear. Your pain-wracked body shouted it out loud and clear, a passionate plea for you to take care of yourself.

"Hey, you! What you're doing in your life is killing me! You're making me work too hard. I can't take it anymore." Ignore this message at your peril, because next time there may be no warning, only the *boom* of the final attack. Do you know that in 55 percent of heart attacks, the first warning sign of a heart attack is *death?*

Those of you who are fortunate enough to survive *must* change your lifestyle. I heard somebody ask "why?" The reason you have to change the way you live is because this lifestyle has already caused *one* heart attack. There is no little insect or reptile that will bite or sting you causing a germ to give you a heart attack. You can't "catch" it from someone at work. I have to assume you didn't particularly like the heart attack you had and do not want another one. If that's the case, then it's time for a change—sometimes a radical change, depending on how far you've pushed the envelope in your life or how close to the edge you live.

Am I saying that change is easy? No, I'm not. Change is extremely difficult. Change takes thought—a lot of thought. Change takes discipline. Change takes desire. And, yes, change takes guts. There is nothing macho about a man who lights up a cigarette (the handsome Marlboro man died of cancer), or swills down that expensive whiskey, or fails to exercise or eat right; nor is it very attractive in women.

Unfortunately, most people don't change much, if at all. Some do. Some very determined, strong-minded, practical individuals change. They succeed in building their bodies back, not only to the place where it was before the heart attack, but to an even healthier level because they are now aware of how precious life and good health can be. They can run marathons, plant flowers, watch their children grow up, and play with their grandchildren and even their great-grandchildren. They can be a joy to all who know and love them. What they have done is maximize the heart's self-healing ability. It's a wonderful organ, designed to keep us alive and kicking for years and years and years.

Chiropractors do not claim to provide treatment for heart conditions—never have, never will. What we do is insure that a patient is free from misaligned vertebrae, which put pressure on the spinal nerves. And what does that pressure do? It interferes with the nerves that run to the heart, the arteries, and the autonomic nervous system, which affects the heart rate, the coronary arteries, and the overall strength of the heart itself.

Even as early as 1921, autopsies on seventy-five cadavers showed that those with diseased hearts had spinal misalignments in the area associated with the nerves that go directly to the heart. The relationship between the spinal column, the spinal nerves, and the cardiovascular system is so intimate and extensive that heart damage can be diagnosed in patients simply by examining the spine.

A number of researchers have also observed that the vertebrae of the middle and lower neck show structural abnormalities in people with heart disease. In another study of 150 cases of various types of heart disease, more than 90 percent showed evidence of spinal abnormalities in the area supplying the heart. Furthermore, three out of four cases showed improvement in the electrocardiogram (EKG) results as well as lowered blood pressure, better sleep habits, and decreased heart damage following chiropractic adjustments and diet and exercise therapy. The other quarter also showed lessened heart muscle damage.

The relatively simple procedure of performing an adjustment to relieve the nerve pressure can actually make the difference between life and death. If you have, or have ever had, heart problems, including heart surgery, you owe it to yourself and those who love you to include chiropractic care as part of your health-care plans.

## Heart Surgery

Medical doctors will be the first to tell you that no surgery is 100-percent safe. Your body's reaction to being cut is extreme. It does not like it. It is a great shock to the body to be exposed to the elements when it has put forth every effort to protect you from such an invasion. Any kind of surgery puts intense stress on the heart. Of the 24.5 million people undergoing surgery every year for noncardiac reasons, 50,000 will suffer heart attacks after surgery, and 20,000 will die from a heart-related problem.

Heart bypass surgery is now performed nearly 300,000 times a year and constitutes a multi-billion dollar industry. It is now considered an established medical practice, thereby qualifying it as legally correct therapy. It is, in my opinion, a money machine.

It is somewhat frightening to learn that one study found that 56 percent of coronary bypass surgeries were done for appropriate reasons. That's more than half. But what about the other 44 percent? Is 56 percent good enough? I don't think so. The same study found that 30 percent were done for "borderline" reasons. In other words, they didn't know what the problem really was or if surgery would help. They just did them anyway. They found that 14 percent were done for inappropriate reasons. How many had to come back for more surgeries? That number was 20 percent. Second bypass operations are four times more dangerous than first operations. Still, are we going to argue with a doctor who tells us that if we don't have this heart surgery, we will not survive? Scare tactics are used every day, and they are *extremely* effective. It is a horrible choice to have to make when you are dealing with your own life—and death.

## WOMEN'S HEALTH

There has been a lot of talk recently about women's health care. Unfortunately, talking about it has been just about all that is being

# *Did You Know...*

. . . that it has been estimated that 30 percent of the 350,000 deaths from coronary heart disease a year (170,000) are caused by smoking?

. . . that nonsmokers who live with smokers have a 20- to 30-percent higher risk of dying from heart disease than do non-smokers who do not live with smokers, making up an estimated 32,000 of heart disease deaths every year?

. . . that four or more cups of coffee a day—regular or decaffeinated—has been shown to increase the risk of heart attacks?

done. The fact that attention is finally being directed toward women's unique health problems is, however, a positive sign.

We are all aware that women are subject to many unique health problems and misconceptions. Even the comedians are having a field day with PMS jokes. The standard medical approach to menstrual complaints has always been controversial. If the doctor is a man, the patient is prone to think that he has no idea what she is talking about. Male doctors have often been accused—and sometimes rightly so—of giving very low priority to ailments specific to women. They dismiss women's complaints about menstrual cramps or other gynecological discomfort as part of the body's normal function. Don't whine about it, they say. Many are simply told to buy drugs off the shelf, while others who have more chronic complaints are given certain prescriptions or surgery. Either way, the *cause* goes untreated and ignored. The woman goes home, takes her Midol, goes to bed with her heating pad for the rest of the day, and keeps her mouth shut about it. After all, it's just Mother Nature's revenge. The curse. Live with it.

## Are All Hysterectomies Necessary?

Do you think all hysterectomies are necessary? Women in the United States are subject to the highest rate of hysterectomy operations in the world—two-and-a-half times the rate of England and four times the rates of Sweden and other European countries. Not only is this operation done on older women, but since 1965 there has been an increase of a whopping 143 percent of hysterectomies done on young women *under thirty years of age.*

The hysterectomy has been called the medical gold mine. It is a frightening thought that these major operations could be done simply to enhance the financial welfare of a medical doctor—but it happens all too often.

Nora W. Coffey, president of HERS Foundation (Hysterectomy Education Resources and Services) believes that hysterectomies are almost always *unnecessary.* "When the ligaments and nerves which attach to the uterus are severed, the anatomical integrity of the pelvis is forever compromised, thus permitting the pelvic and hip bones to gradually widen," she said. "Naturally, this changes the alignment of the entire skeleton, often resulting in lower back, hip, and knee pain."

Further observations of hysterectomy patients show that they experience urinary incontinence, bowel problems, diminished blood flow, bone and joint pain, memory loss, depression, a profound loss of stamina and sex drive, and many other physical and emotional problems. Seldom are the patients warned about these all-too-common problems.

How many men do you know who have had their penises surgically removed—not counting those on the daytime talk shows? Yet medical doctors routinely cut out the female sexual organs. They often call this surgery *preventative.* If you were moving to Alaska, would you have your fingers and toes amputated to *prevent* them from being frostbitten?

If the doctor warns his or her patients about all the problems that go along with surgery, preventative or otherwise, he or she will not collect the fee for the operation should the patient wisely decide against the surgery. The other scenario is that the doctor honestly does not know—was never taught in medical school—about even the possibility of these problems!

According to Ms. Coffey, the hysterectomy is one of the most commonly performed surgical procedures in the country, second only to the Caesarean section. As proof of how often this operation is needlessly performed, the HERS Foundation referred 16,000 women who were told that they needed a hysterectomy to gynecologists who specialized in the conditions for which the hysterectomy was prescribed. Of these women, 90 percent were told that they did not need a hysterectomy and were treated otherwise. Many did not require any treatment at all.

We are not saying that a hysterectomy is *never* necessary. With severe infection of the reproductive organs; dead tissue in the uterus; and cancer of the cervix, uterus, or ovaries that will not respond to more conservative care, there may be no other alternative but surgery. The key, again, is to seek alternatives and educate yourself about your choices. Ms. Coffey believes that the procedure should have been abandoned in the Dark Ages, yet it continues to be performed on close to one million women every year. Have we another big medical money machine here?

## Menopause

There are still some medical doctors who consider menopause a disease rather than a normal physiologic state. Drug therapies for menopause are commonplace, instead of the exploration of more natural healing approaches. Dangerous side effects may often result from these drug therapies.

The relationship between the female reproductive system, nervous system, endocrine (or hormonal) system, and the spinal column is extremely important. The nervous system and the hormonal system work together to ensure that the ovaries, Fallopian tubes, uterus, cervix, vagina, and related structures function normally. Drug therapy can alter this balance. Many women are not aware that organs other than the sexual organs are responsible for the health of the reproductive system. Chemicals produced by the ovaries and adrenals (small glands situated on top of the kidneys) that are essential for reproduction are deactivated, or broken down, by the liver. If the liver is not functioning correctly (which could happen as a result of drug therapy), these chemicals can build up to an unhealthy level and cause fibroid tumors in the uterus, which, although benign, account for at least one-third of all gynecological admissions to the hospitals.

## Chiropractic and Women's Health

Chiropractic has been a blessing to countless women with various reproductive problems, including the dreaded and much maligned premenstrual syndrome (PMS). Many women who suffer from menstrual cramps also suffer from spinal problems such as back pain. Chiropractors understand the relationship between the spine, lower back, and the female anatomy. We believe that subluxations allow the gynecological problems to happen in the first place. We believe there is a direct cause/symptom relationship here.

In one study of 122 women, the majority of dysmenorrhea (painful menstruation) sufferers had lower back problems and spinal displacements. This is why many women who visit a chiropractor because of their back pain report beneficial effects from menstrual cramps as well as other gynecological problems. These are the kind of "side effects" all women should encounter.

Scientific investigation into the relationship between spinal health and gynecological problems has reported encouraging, and sometimes amazing, results. In a 1973 study of 496 patients who received spinal care, more than 95 percent experienced relief of general gynecological problems. A 1986 study found spinal care to have a beneficial effect on PMS in particular. In 1990, another study found that "dysfunction of the uterus and structural fixation of the same spinal segments of innervation can be indicative of a somatovisceral reflex. . . . Adjusting these vertebrae and creating motion in the joints seemed to influence the exiting nerves, restoring proper nervous transmission to the uterus."

## Should Pregnant Women Go to a Chiropractor?

Pregnant women should *absolutely* go to a chiropractor! Have you ever known of a mother-to-be who does not at one time or another during her pregnancy, complain of her back hurting—especially in the final stages? Since chiropractic care is a method of keeping the body free from spinal nerve stress by ensuring that the spinal column is functioning properly, what better time for a woman to have this care than when another life is entrusted to her?

A pregnant woman needs to have her body as healthy and strong as possible in order to handle pregnancy and childbirth. Chiropractic care will help insure that the reproductive system and other systems so essential for a healthy pregnancy will receive an uninterrupted nerve supply from the spinal column. During this time in her life the slightest interference or stress to the nerve supply could adversely affect the baby, as well as the mother.

Most expectant mothers know that it is best to remain completely drug-free during pregnancy. Since chiropractic is a drugless health-care system, it is an ideal alternative to those types of drugs and medications that have been linked to fetal damage or malformations. I find it hard to believe how often medical doctors are still prescribing medicine to pregnant women. All drugs have side effects, and the medication the mother takes directly affects the baby as well. Could this be the reason that the United States ranks only twentieth in the world in keeping our babies alive?

Women probably worry more during this period of their lives than at any other time because their concern is not for themselves alone. They are concerned about carrying the baby to full term, having a healthy baby, morning sickness, backaches, leg pain, and a safe and easy delivery.

Can we help to alleviate any of these worries in the chiropractor's office? We certainly can. We know from firsthand experience that this is true, and an article written by K. Stein that appeared in the July 1964 issue of the *ACA* (American Chiropractic Association) *Journal of Chiropractic* entitled, "The Value of Chiropractic Care in Cases of Pregnancy," underscores this fact. "Chiropractic care during pregnancy can help women in their ability to become pregnant and maintain pregnancy, in controlling vomiting during pregnancy, in delivering full-term infants with ease, and producing infants healthier than the normal population."

Chiropractors are trained in adjusting the spines of pregnant women, and most chiropractic adjusting tables have special modifications for the pregnant figure. It is safe, not only for her, but for her unborn baby as well. Besides, where else can a woman lay on her stomach when she is in her eighth month of pregnancy?

I'm often asked how late into pregnancy can an adjustment be done, and I point out that there have been patients who have received adjustments even during labor. There are reported cases of a chiropractor being called in to perform a spinal adjustment when labor had ceased. Immediately after the adjustments are made, the woman's labor resumed.

If there is one conclusion I hope you will draw from this portion of the book, it is this: A healthy spinal column is essential for the health of the female reproductive system. It is also vital for women, with or without gynecological problems, to get routine spinal checkups by a doctor of chiropractic as regularly as she keeps her regular medical or dentist appointments.

## INFECTIONS AND INFLAMMATION

I wish there were enough time and space to discuss all the illnesses and disabilities that chiropractic care can relieve, but, unfortunately, I must draw the line somewhere. There are a few others, however, that I would like to discuss briefly at this time.

All people, healthy and otherwise, are filled with germs. You would think we'd all be sick all the time, but our bacteria-filled bodies are quite normal. We actually develop the diseases that have been inhabiting our bodies for some time, when something goes haywire in our immune system (see Chapter 5).

The medical establishment has certain ways to destroy infections. We sometimes take antibiotics that may help at the time, but the infection may come back later. The overuse of antibiotics has, unfortunately, created an antibiotic-resistant strain of "supergerms" causing millions of "superinfections." Hospital-acquired infections are responsible for between 50,000 and 100,000 deaths every year. Also, there are 2 million patients who "catch" hospital-acquired infections every year that cause them to have to remain in the hospital for an average of seven extra days.

We know that taking an antibiotic for a cold is useless—still they are prescribed. There are times when antibiotics and other drugs can be life-saving, when used appropriately. This is why we need to be educated thoroughly about our own bodies and what harm can come to them by medications that destroy rather than heal.

Hippocrates said that "inflammation is the flame which cleanses the body." Inflammation is one of the body's most powerful forms of cleansing and healing. It usually manifests itself as heat, redness, swelling, and, most often, pain. It can be found in conditions ranging from a pesky insect bite to pneumonia.

When your child wakes up in the night, sick to her stomach, the vomiting or diarrhea that often accompanies the illness is her body's way of discharging the intruders from her system. When the body wants to eliminate that which it does not want—or is causing distress—it usually does so without ceremony. Afterwards, the child will feel better, look better, and act better. Illnesses such as sore throats, chicken pox, and earaches usually heal themselves within a short period of time. Others, such as allergic and autoimmune diseases like asthma, rheumatic diseases, and chronic skin problems, may take a long time—or may never completely disappear.

If inflammations are helped to work themselves out of the body, they will usually heal with time. It is those inflammations that are treated by pushing them back into the body—the way most medical treatments work—that may never heal. They may go away temporarily, but they will return, usually in some new or more debilitating form, causing many other seemingly unrelated symptoms.

Today, the diseases of modern civilization—heart disease, stroke, cancer, and emphysema—are the main causes of adult death. The question we must ask is this: Can it be that these chronic diseases of adulthood result from the suppression of inflammatory diseases in our childhood?

The answer may very well be in the affirmative.

The Foundation for Advance of Cancer Therapy in Philadelphia reached the following conclusion in 1991: "The inappropriate use of antibiotics and other suppressive drugs, as well as the excessive use of immunizations, are some of the biggest factors in the increase in chronic disease and cancer that we're seeing in modern countries, in adults as well as children."

Chiropractic treatment is expressive in nature. It respects the natural healing process of the body. Sometimes a patient who seeks chiropractic care for inflammation may, at first, experience an even higher fever along with vomiting, discharge, diarrhea, and other increased symptoms of elimination and cleansing after the adjustment. It is this method of getting rid of problems that helps the body rejuvenate itself enough to heal properly in a *natural* way. Periodic cleansing and detoxifying are infinitely more healthy than weakening, aging, and poisoning the body with medical cures.

## ALLERGIES

Does it seem to you that almost every little baby born today suffers from some kind of allergy? Some are not much more than an aggravation, while others can be literally life-threatening.

There are endless varieties of allergies, most of which are impossible not only to diagnose but to "cure" as well. The causes of allergies and immune system disease have not been conclusively determined, but there are some who feel strongly that childhood vaccinations lay the foundation for autoimmune diseases and other disorders of the immune system. Orthodox medicine has no cure for allergies—only treatment, most of which is less than satisfactory, and sometimes worse than the problem itself. Millions of patients have received allergy shots over the past fifty years, but there are no long-term studies to determine possible neurologic or other types of consequences of this rather experimental treatment.

The September 1989 issue of *The American Chiropractor* cites a three-year study of 107 individuals who had been under chiropractic care for five years or more. The chiropractic patients "were found to have 200 percent greater immune competence than people who had not received chiropractic care and 400 percent greater immune competence than people with cancer and other serious diseases. The superiority of those under chiropractic care did not diminish with age!"

All illnesses are upsetting in the least and deadly at the worst. We know that allergies can make life miserable for some people. The short-term method of relief offered by the medical profession is both controversial and dangerous, and its long-term effects are untested. Sometimes plain old common sense needs to prevail. Often recommended is a twofold approach. One, to avoid, if possible, those substances that cause severe reactions; and two, to correct the basic cause, which is the malfunction of your immune system.

K. W. Donsback points out in the article "Allergies," that "a healthy body is capable of neutralizing those toxic substances, and a body which has malfunctioning defense mechanisms cannot. The emphasis on allergies must be on building a healthy body, not on trying to use evasive tactics by eliminating all the allergens."

It would also help if our air were cleaner, all of our food were grown organically, and we avoided all toxic substances. But since that is unlikely, we have to take some control to help our bodies to do the best job that they can do.

## DIGESTIVE DISORDERS

Americans spend $1,369,863 *every day* on laxatives. Does it help? Evidently not. We still suffer from all those digestive disorders. Colitis, an inflammation of the colon, is the most common of all digestive disorders, affecting 15 to 20 percent of all Americans.

Diverticulosis and diverticulitis are problems suffered by almost half of Americans over the age of forty. Most people with diverticulosis are totally unaware of their problem. *Diverticulosis* is the presence of diverticula (pouchlike bulges in the muscular wall) in the intestines, particularly the colon. It is only when diverticulosis becomes *diverticulitis* (an inflamed diverticulum) that it becomes painfully evident. Symptoms include severe abdominal cramping (usually on the lower left side) fever, nausea, constipation, diarrhea, and/or rectal bleeding. Bed rest and lots of liquids are often prescribed to rest the colon in cases of diverticulitis. In some cases where there are a number of diverticula, there may be a need for their surgical removal to lower the risk of inflammation. In rare cases, an infected diverticulum can rupture and cause life-threatening *peritonitis,* or blood poisoning, requiring emergency surgery.

Colon cancer strikes 110,000 people every year and kills over 53,000. Contributors to this illness are inactivity and a high-fat, low-fiber diet (the opposite of what is recommended for general good health). Studies have shown that those who lead even moderately physically active lives cut the risk of colon cancer in half.

Another illness that strikes half of people over forty is hemorrhoids. Though hemorrhoids are usually not found *in* the digestive system, they are often the result of problems of it. Now this may be another subject for comedians, but those who suffer from this affliction are not amused. Hemorrhoids are swollen veins around the anus that are very sensitive and painful and may bleed or even protrude outside the body. Hemorrhoids affect those who suffer from constipation or diarrhea or those experiencing increased abdominal pressure from pregnancy, chronic coughing, or very strenuous work or exercise. Many prescribed drugs may actually cause the condition to worsen, some even causing gastrointestinal bleeding. Medical treatments generally prescribed for external hemorrhoids are usually creams or ointments that often contain anesthetics and hydrocortisone. Surgery is sometimes recommended in extreme cases.

Many still want that "magic bullet," something to make everything all right without having to contribute anything to that end. That's one reason why medicine is so popular. You really don't have to do anything but pop a pill or allow yourself to be put to sleep on an operating table while somebody else does the work.

As far as I know, life has no magic bullet. We must continue to watch what we eat—which includes educating ourselves about the best and worst of food choices—we must exercise, and we must be under regular preventative chiropractic care. Lack of proper diet and reasonable exercise, and abusive lifestyles are major culprits in the causes of cardiovascular disease, cancer, and other chronic illnesses.

If I listed all the problems chiropractic addresses, you would shake your head in disbelief. But the fact is that while chiropractic does not claim to *treat* any of our health problems, it does help the best "physician" heal those diseases. Your body is still your best friend and doctor when it comes to illness, serious or otherwise.

We as a populace are, unfortunately, not getting healthier. We are getting sicker and we need a change. We need a natural health-care system, nontoxic treatments, and an overall educational concept of what good health really is.

We need chiropractic health care.

# Chapter 9

# No Bad Babies

*When Art Linkletter was once asked about his favorite interview with children, he gave an amusing, yet insightful example.*

*The children were chosen for his show, he explained, not by the show's producers, nor by him, but by their teachers. When Linkletter asked one little first-grader why he thought the teacher selected him for the show, the boy did not hesitate for a moment.*

*"I'm the smartest kid in the class," he said with innocent candor.*

*"Did your teacher tell you that?" Linkletter asked, trying to suppress a smile.*

*"No," the child answered. "I noticed it myself."*

Children, if the natural order of things were followed, would come into the world knowing they were the finest and most wonderful example of God's handiwork. And as they grew, they would continue to hold this belief, because it is the truth.

The world does not always welcome a child with open arms, and, unfortunately, many are told through harsh treatment or neglect that they are of little value. Sometimes even the best of us, through ignorance or thoughtlessness, are guilty of failing to give these precious little ones the proper start in life.

"What a dumb thing you did!"

"You are stupid."

"You don't have a brain in your head."

"What's wrong with you?"
"You'll never amount to anything."
"You don't do anything right."
"You're bad!"

The little boy on Linkletter's show, however, was convinced of his worth, and I'm sure that not only was he happy with himself, but he was a healthy, well cared for little person as well.

## MY FIRST CHILD

I can remember vividly when my first child, Steven, was born. Like most new fathers, I was a little hesitant around him at first. He was so new, so small, and seemed so fragile. I recall being very happy he had finally arrived; and to give you an indication of how little most new parents know, I actually thought his arrival would make my life a little easier. I welcomed him with an almost selfish relief. As we had gone through the nine months of waiting—and trust me, it was not only trying for the mother, but for me as well—I was more than ready for this to be over and done with. Actually, it was just beginning. But my first thought was, "Now we can relax." Yeah, right!

It was at this point that a very unusual thing happened. We had been told by other parents, and, of course, we had read in all those books expectant parents read, that this new person would dramatically affect our lives. During the waiting period, we knew this in theory, but it was not until he arrived that we knew it in absolute reality.

I soon realized that my life would never be the same again. I would never have the feeling I once had—the freedom nor the peace of mind. Now, that is not a negative statement, but a true concept of parenthood. When a child comes into your life, you realize that you have someone who is completely dependent upon you and that you are in total control of this tiny human being's life, his present and his future. While the baby is in the mother, you have a built-in baby sitter. But as soon as the child is born, reality hits you right between the eyes.

Add to this the heart-stopping fear that something might happen, that something might go wrong with the baby, and you have a very heavy load suddenly cast upon your shoulders—and your heart. I remember walking into Steven's room many, many times just to watch him, to make sure his little chest was rising and falling as he slept. I had to see if he was still actually breathing. It's extremely scary because I knew, maybe even better than some other parents, how few of the answers we really know.

Babies have a tendency to take away some of your smugness and arrogance. It took me only a short time to find out that it is a lot easier to give advice to others when it is not your child you're talking about. I also realized that from here on, I would have to give a big part of my life, every day, to this new person. That, alone, is an awesome responsibility. Selfishness would now have to be replaced by selflessness if I were going to be a good parent.

I also knew I would have to make the right and proper decisions for his own good until he was old enough to do this on his own. In court cases we often hear the term "in the best interest of the child," and it is not until you look into the face of one of these precious little people that you realize exactly what that profound statement is all about. Furthermore, there is no amount of education, no number of impressive degrees that will prepare you for this unique and challenging position. It's strange how we have to be certified to work on an automobile or trained to arrange flowers at a florist or flip hamburgers at McDonalds, but we are not required to know anything or undergo any training to be a parent. Although there are many good books available and even places where you can take parenting classes, there is no Parenting 101 course in college that I am aware of. They don't make you take a test in order to take your baby home from the hospital. Somehow we are just supposed to know how to be a good parent.

As the child grows, we also know that others will be watching our every move. They will observe our attitudes and methods of raising a child. I have to ask myself as well what are my goals and desires for this child? Which road will I select for him? How will I prepare him to choose that which is right? What will be the results of my efforts?

There is no doubt that there is no greater responsibility (or joy) than having a child. We are never absolutely 100-percent positive about what is really best for our kids, but I would like to believe that we all want our children to have the very best opportunity to grow up to be happy and healthy people. Unfortunately, I know through my experience and observations as a doctor that some parents do not share this opinion, and in some cases, should never have become parents at all. For those of us who are thrilled with the joy that being a parent brings, we find it almost impossible to understand those who not only don't want the children they have brought into the world but cause these innocent little ones great physical and mental anguish that will almost surely affect them, even into their adult lives, perpetuating itself in their children and in their children's children.

This chapter is for those of us who want what is best for our children and want to bring them up in a loving home as free of pain, sickness, and dis-ease as possible. Being a parent, especially nowadays, is very difficult. It is not a walk in the park. It is a wonderful journey, however, filled with lots of decisions, lots of pressures, lots of advice, lots of wonder, lots of pain, lots of joy, and endless choices.

Parenthood is not for sissies.

## BABY STEPS TO HEALTH

In my office there is a sign that begins with "Leave your children at home . . ." and at first glance some people might think that I don't like children—that they would be distracting if brought to my office. Nothing could be further from the truth. Not only do I love children and have never considered them a bother or a distraction, but I believe the one place they really belong is in a chiropractor's office. The rest of the sign says, " . . . *so they can suffer the way you have for the rest of their lives.*" What the sign means is bring your children in to have their spines checked.

You're not serious—I can hear some of you saying. Yes, I am. I'm very serious. Some people are aghast at the thought of having a small child adjusted. Yet these same people think nothing of pumping the same child full of drugs and subjecting them to shots and all kinds of chemicals that can do them irreparable harm—sometimes even causing death.

## THE COMMON COLD—UNCOMMON CURES

What happens in most households when little Amanda starts coming down with the sniffles? Quick, run to the medicine cabinet and start giving her some pills or liquids or lozenges. It's what a good mother or father does, isn't it? We would think so because we've been programmed to think that. Especially with all the television commercials promoting different types of medications, we would tend to believe they would be the right answer for our children's ailments.

However, maybe there is hope because the tide seems to be changing somewhat. This change is long overdue. Parents are asking more questions today, seeking better answers, and checking into alternative health-care methods. Furthermore, there are now articles in national magazines and newspapers as well as features on television shows that not only point out the dangers of accepting all that is prescribed for our children but warn us to beware.

I was very encouraged to note a page-one article in the October 5, 1994 issue of *USA Today* addressing the problem of parents giving over-the-counter drugs to preschool children for the treatment of colds, despite potential for harm. The article stated that there is little proof that the drugs are effective in combating the illness.

The article, which was based on an article taken from *The Journal of the American Medical Association*, gives the results of a survey made by the National Center for Health Statistics. The survey, which was conducted with 8,145 mothers of 3-year-old children, found 53.7 percent of the children had been given an over-the-counter drug in the previous thirty days—usually various cold medicines and painkillers.

The survey went on to confirm that 70 percent of the children with a recent illness received over-the-counter drugs, and half had been given two types of drugs. The study showed that white, married, educated mothers with good incomes were most likely to give drugs to their children. Dr. Michael Weintraub of the Food and Drug Administration, was also quoted as saying that, although side effects from these cold medicines are *generally* not serious, the potential is there for adverse reactions and oversedation.

It is easy for a good parent to want to do something for a sick child. Nothing distresses us more than the helpless feeling of watching our little ones suffer. Dr. Ann Gadomski of the University of Maryland says that this is why parents "become easy prey to . . . promotion by the drug companies."

It should be a warning to all of us to learn that from 1985 through 1989, there were 670,000 reports made to poison control centers involving over-the-counter drugs in children under the age of six.

In conclusion, the study came up with the finding that most of the upper respiratory tract infections among preschoolers are caused by viruses, and there is no cure for these infections. It is like that old-fashioned "cure for the cold"—with medicine you can stop it in seven days, but without medication it may take as long as a week.

I never underestimate the concern and sometimes panic of a parent, especially new ones, when a child is ill. We had that experience with Steven. Unfortunately, my wife had the flu when he was born, and what normally might have been an inconvenience became a major problem. Without my knowledge, our newborn was given a shot of antibiotics that was supposed to prevent him from getting sick. This is what the medical community considers prevention. What this did, instead, was weaken his little immune system, leaving him extremely vulnerable to all kinds of other monsters, including many viruses. He was a sitting duck for whatever bug came along.

Christmas—and with it, numerous relatives—soon came, and of course, one of them had a virus with symptoms of fever, aches, congestion, and a wicked cough. Steven, who was only six weeks old at the time, caught it immediately. Needless to say, we were extremely alarmed because we had a very sick baby. They don't make a Hallmark Christmas ornament that would depict "Baby's First Christmas" at our house that year. We had to watch him around the clock. There were several nights when his breathing was so labored that we would take him into the bathroom, turn on all the hot water, and let the steam help open him up.

I couldn't understand how he had gotten so sick. I had done everything I knew of to help him strengthen his immune system. I checked his spine within minutes of his birth. My wife,

Debbie, was breast-feeding him and carefully monitoring what she ate. We hadn't taken him out to the malls or into any kind of crowds. In fact, we had been so careful, we were totally frustrated that he had become so sick so quickly. This really disturbed me—not only that it had happened—but the mystery of the reason *why* it happened. I was still unaware of the antibiotic he had received shortly after his birth. Debbie happened to mention "the shot" one day when we were talking.

"What shot?" I asked. "He's never had a shot."

She then vaguely recalled that while she was still groggy after Steven's birth, the doctor came into the room and said she wanted to give the baby a shot of antibiotics. The shot had, in my opinion, totally wiped out his immune system. If I had known he'd had the shot, I would have protected him better from contact with people until his immune system had time to recover.

We continued using all the natural methods we knew of to help him regain his own health, with the help of his own small body and his weakened immune system. It took a good five weeks before he really got over being sick (and being doctored), but fortunately, he was much stronger afterwards. His immune system was rejuvenated, and he has been an extremely healthy child ever since. I believe that had he not been given the shot right after his birth, he would not have become sick in the first place. Medical doctors give out antibiotics so freely, it borders on carelessness. I just wonder how many times this scenario still happens. It is very unfortunate that people who do not understand how the body works allow their child to be given more and more antibiotics causing a continuing cycle of sickness—antibiotics—sickness—antibiotics—sickness—antibiotics, leaving them with no idea why their baby stays stick and can't get rid of the colds, fevers, and ear infections.

## CHIROPRACTIC AND YOUR BABY

All infants, as well as adults, need a healthy spinal column. Nobody disagrees with that. But most people don't understand that it is quite possible that their baby did not make it into the world with a well-aligned spinal column. It may at the time seem like no big thing because the baby is no big thing, but the trauma of birth could—and often does—cause physical injury to the baby.

The beginning of all life takes place with a tiny brain cell, which expands into the spinal cord, and then into the rest of the nervous system. Our entire being is centered around the spinal column and the nervous system. Think about that wonderful comfort the unborn baby feels inside the womb. Then, a world of darkness, warmth, softness, and quiet gives way to a harsh, cold, blinding world of noise and confusion. The baby is brutally separated from his or her mother, often dangled from its heels and whacked across the rear. Welcome to the real world! (And to poor spinal alignment.)

Many studies have shown that the majority of newborns have spinal nerve stress that is both health- and life-threatening. The birth process is a potentially traumatic and sometimes crippling event for the baby. The obstetrical manipulation, and even the application of standard orthodox procedures, can sometimes prove intolerable for the baby. It has been noted also that most signs of neonatal injury observed in the delivery room are neurological. Childbirth, which is a naturally occurring event, has been turned into a major surgical procedure. Unfortunately, most procedures are done to suit the ease, desires, and whims of the doctor, but not those of the mother or the baby. It's unfortunate, but too many times I've been told by a mother that during childbirth, the doctor was pulling so forcefully on the baby that she felt herself being pulled forward on the table. Childbirth was not supposed to be so difficult for the mother or so traumatic for the baby. All in all, childbirth is the final product of an act of love and should be treated with love. Childbirth is about new life. It's about hope. It's about a new beginning. Yet because of the way it's handled, we have far too many injuries and too much trauma, pain, and unhappiness. It is supposed to be a positive act, but it turns into something negative.

Many doctors will tell you how resilient these little people are, and, amazingly enough, they are. But they can, and often do, suffer from the trauma of poor birthing methods. Others will argue that babies do not suffer from spinal trauma. Don't bet the farm—or your child's good health—on it. Of course they can suffer from spinal trauma. Those delicate little bodies can certainly be thrown out of kilter, so it's imperative that you have them checked by a chiropractor as soon as possible after birth.

Chiropractors believe that our bodies possess an inborn natural wisdom that will work for you if there is no interference. If a birth takes place in the most natural position and is done without drugs or intervention of any kind (unless absolutely necessary) you have a better chance of having a healthy baby. God knew the best way, don't you think?

There have been many studies done concerning child care in the chiropractic health centers, but one stands out as a fine example. In an article in the German medical journal *Manuelle Medizin*, authors Guttmann and Fyrmann reported examining a random group of 1,250 babies five days after their birth. The report showed that 211 suffered from vomiting, hyperactivity, and sleeplessness. Spinal abnormalities in 95 percent of this group were revealed through manual examination. It was also discovered that spinal adjustment "frequently resulted in immediate quieting, cessation of crying, muscular relaxation, and sleepiness."

The writers also noted that spinal nerve stress in the upper neck causes "many clinical features, from central motor impairment to lower resistance to infection—especially ear, nose, and throat infections." It is also their consensus that a spinal check-up should be obligatory after every birth—especially difficult births.

One 18-month-old baby boy in the study suffered from tonsillitis, frequent enteritis, therapy-resistant conjunctivitis, frequent colds, earache, and increased problems getting to sleep. In short, the child was a cranky, crying, sickly baby that drove the parents to wonder what they were doing wrong, or if something was seriously wrong with the child. After one spinal adjustment, the child was put to bed where he "slept like a baby" until morning. The removal of nerve interference allowed his body to start the healing process.

A major modern miracle? No, it was simply a routine chiropractic adjustment for a child whose parents were searching for something to help their child. Unfortunately, people usually don't bring their children to a chiropractor early. We get the really chronic, sickly, weakened children who have already taken lots of drugs and been to many doctors but received little or no help. We usually don't get the easy problems, yet we get more and more kids every day through word of mouth. That's why I'm writing this book. For far too long, chiropractors have allowed the medical profession to push us around. We haven't really said what we believe because of fear of retaliation. We've tried to melt into mainstream medicine and health care because we think that's what the people want.

We are still misunderstood by many people and we have done a poor job of teaching the public what chiropractic is all about, especially when it comes to children. Chiropractors are different from medical doctors, and we should be proud of it. We should work to maintain that difference. Fortunately, our patients have no problem at all extoling the benefits of chiropractic.

A prime example of the benefits of chiropractic care for children is the story of one of my patients, Glen Motz, and his daughter. When his oldest daughter, Veronica, was brought home from the hospital, she would not (or could not) sleep. She was fine in an upright position, but as soon as they laid her down to put her to sleep, she would start crying. This went on for about six months. Their pediatrician was of little help. He made suggestions, but nothing worked. I finally convinced Glen to bring the baby in for an adjustment. From the day of her first adjustment on, Veronica slept through the night. Coincidence? I don't think so.

It's patients like Glen and his family that help me realize how important this war against dis-ease is and how people really need to be told the true, unedited chiropractic story. When it comes to the health of our children, we need to be on guard to give them the best possible start in life, as well as health maintenance care. Chiropractic is not just the natural approach to good health—it's the *only* approach to continuing good health.

As mentioned earlier, today's hospitals utilize birthing methods that make the process easier for the doctor but more difficult for the mother and child. Earlier methods utilized midwives and birthing stools, allowing for a more natural delivery. Today the doctor often has to pull, stretch, and twist the infant's body to bring him or her into the world. Fortunately, the seriousness of spinal injuries at birth is now more widely recognized. Harvard University pathologist Dr. Abraham Towbin reported that spinal cord and brain stem injury is present in up to 33 percent of newborn deaths. This translates into 20,000 infant fatalities a year in this country alone.

Dr. Towbin believes that mechanical stress imposed by obstetrical manipulation—even the application of standard orthodox procedures—may prove to be intolerable for the baby. He wrote that "forceful longitudinal traction during delivery, particularly when combined with flexion and torsion of the vertebral axis, is thought to be the most important cause of neonatal spinal injury."

## Are Adjustments Traumatic for Children?

Chiropractic is not traumatic for children. All infants need a healthy spinal column. A checkup by a doctor of chiropractic to check for the presence of vertebral subluxations or spinal nerve stress may save your child a lifetime of pain or discomfort. It just may also save your child's life. I might point out at this time that a chiropractic adjustment for a child is not the same as an adjustment for an adult. A spinal adjustment given a baby is very gentle—so gentle that if the baby happened to be sleeping, it would not even awaken him or her. Children are very easy to work with because their problems haven't been there very long. The freedom of motion allows us to do our job with little or no effort. As a chiropractor, I simply give the baby a little help to do what his or her body is already programmed to do. The baby's own innate intelligence makes him or her want to be in the right position, and in many ways the child actually helps the chiropractor do his or her job without realizing it.

Sometimes, if the baby is healthy, his or her spine will straighten without adjustments, but, unfortunately, that's not always the case. An unhealthy spine can interfere with the normal function of the nervous system and may cause serious health problems, both during infancy and throughout the child's life. We've all seen those newborns that can't seem to adjust to the world around them. They are always crying ("just a little colic"), or won't stand for the parent to lay them down ("spoiled rotten"), or simply cannot be placated in any way ("a difficult child"), and sometimes these patterns set the pace for the child's entire life.

Famed animal behavior specialist Barbara Woodhouse wrote a best seller entitled *No Bad Dogs* in which she lays the blame of a dog's misbehavior at the feet of the trainer and/or the owner. With children, much more than discipline and training is involved. A healthy child is much easier to discipline. A healthy child gives little grief to his or her parents or others. A healthy child likes him- or herself and others. A healthy self-esteem is much more difficult to attain when one is in poor physical health. Babies do not know that it is not normal to feel pain or discomfort. They only know how to express their pain by crying. Even older children who have always been sickly do not realize that this is not normal. In time, when they come to realize that it is not normal to be so sick, they may come to think this burden is their fault, and they must somehow be different. Hence, poor self-esteem, poor grades in school, and poor social skills equal an overall miserable kid that most people would rather not be around—spoiled, rotten brat.

I fully believe there are "No Bad Babies," only children whose health problems are controlling their lives, and, unfortunately, will continue to do so. The little boy on Linkletter's show *noticed* himself that he was smart. Further questions would probably have brought out the facts that he noticed that he was loved as well. This is not to say that unhealthy children aren't loved. They are. They are loved sometimes to the point of overcompensation, and as a result, may suffer even more and still not know why. Sadly enough, neither does the parent.

## Why Don't Medical Doctors Notice the Need for a Baby's Spine to Be Adjusted?

Medical doctors are trained to intervene—to take charge when something appears to be *wrong*. Prevention, whether dealing with adults or children, is not a top priority in our health-care system. Some of our most respected chiropractors and medical doctors hold the belief that obstetricians constantly interfere in a natural physiological process and that they insist on treating childbirth as though it were a disease. It is a shocking thought

# Did You Know...

... that many forms of alternative medicine are considered effective for treating chronic diseases in Europe? European countries are not behind us, rather they are ahead in the acceptance of complementary, alternative, or nontoxic health-care methods, which have been used for many years throughout Europe by medical and nonmedical doctors. These methods include: body detoxification, fresh juice fasting, colonics, spinal manipulation, reflexology massage, and herbal and homeopathic remedies.

that medical interference with a normal bodily function can adversely affect the physical or intellectual capacity of a child for the rest of his or her life. Sometimes it even ends that life before it really has a chance to begin. Hospital births expose the baby to an array of obstetrical hazards—yet fear of the unknown will certainly keep some parents from trying home birth. Having your baby at home is less risky than going to the hospital because much of the most dangerous technology employed in hospitals is not available to doctors or midwives who deliver babies at home. Procedures such as the use of ultrasound; internal fetal monitoring; and excessive use of sedatives, pain relievers, Caesarean section, and induced labor are, for the most part, avoided when the mother delivers her baby at home.

Parents are sometimes shocked to discover that many studies show home birth to be safer for both mother and child. Lewis E. Mehl, M.D., of the University of Wisconsin Infant Development Center reviewed 1,000 births, nearly half of which had taken place at home, and came up with the following findings:

- There were thirty birth injuries among the hospital-born children and none among those born at home.

- Fifty-two of the babies born in the hospital required resuscitation, versus only fourteen of those born at home.

- Six hospital babies suffered neurological damage compared with one born at home.

If you choose to have your baby in a hospital, and there is trauma connected with the birth (and this can also happen at home to a lesser degree); the best thing you can do for your baby as soon as you get home is take him or her to a chiropractor and have his or her spinal column checked.

## Chiropractic and Learning Disabilities

While it's true that we still need to know a great deal more about what spinal nerve stress does to an infant, we know enough to realize that we should pay a lot more attention to the problem. Learning and behavioral problems can also be connected to spinal nerve stress and can sometimes be too subtle to be tested. The bottom line is that the difference between an exceptional child and an average or below-average child may be traced to a spinal misalignment. Why take any chances?

Studies have shown that learning disabilities can indeed be helped by chiropractic care. Personally, I am a strong believer in trying this method before subjecting any child to mind-altering drugs and medications. Standard medications are notorious for their terrible side effects. You've heard the old saying that the cure is worse than the disease—well, that's not too far off. Chiropractic health care can be an alternative to the chemical route of Ritalin and other such medications, and I am not alone in that opinion.

In 1972, the Psychoeducational and Guidance Service, working with the Texas State Chiropractic Association, agreed to refer some students for chiropractic care to see if it would improve their ability to learn. The twenty-four students selected were periodically evaluated as part of the research program. Half of the students received chiropractic care, and half were treated with medication.

The conclusion of the study was that ". . . Chiropractic treatment was more effective for the wide-range symptoms common in the neurological dysfunction syndrome in which thirteen symptoms or problem areas were considered." The report went on to say, "Statistically, the chiropractic treatment was 20 to 40 percent more effective than the commonly used medications." Based on this study, and from what I have experienced personally with my patients, it is apparent that a child taken to a chiropractor and checked on a regular basis is less likely to develop problems in the first place.

There is no way to describe the sense of satisfaction derived from watching a young mind discover its potential. If I had a child who was faced with learning disabilities, I would not hesitate to seek an alternative to the drug route. I believe we can work with the child's psychologists and school counselors and take a far more active role in helping these often misunderstood children through this problem.

In his book *Adjustments (The Making of a Chiropractor)*, Vincent T. Joseph, D.C., wrote about one of his patients who came to his office one day in tears. She told him that school officials were going to take her son Alexander out of school because he was learning disabled, and the teacher could not handle him. When asked what kinds of tests had been done on the boy, the mother said they had not done any tests yet. The *teacher* had simply "diagnosed" his problems on her own and wanted him put on Ritalin. The mother admitted that there had been more than a few problems with him, both at school and at home, but she was terrified to use Ritalin.

Like most parents of children who are learning disabled, Alex's mother did not know the side effects of Ritalin, such as permanent learning disabilities, stunted growth, loss of appetite, and many more equally frightening symptoms. Many doctors fail to do proper exams and give little thought to alternatives such as chiropractic care, change of diet, or other simple, "old-fashioned" preventative measures. Our society has made it too easy (and too acceptable) to just "pop a pill" for instant results.

Dr. Joseph concurred that there may be a place for Ritalin, but not without exhausting all other alternatives first. There should be a professional and thorough diagnosis of the child's problems before any drug is considered.

Alex had been tested at school, and, as expected, he failed all of the tests. He was way behind in motor skills, mathematical skill level—everything. His mother suspected that the teacher, who insisted the boy could not function without Ritalin, simply didn't like him and wanted him drugged into submissiveness. The teacher refused to have Alex in her class if he was not on the drug.

"What does he eat?" was the first question Dr. Joseph asked

the mother. The reply included the staples of the basic childhood diet—hot dogs, hamburgers, pizza, macaroni and cheese,
fried chicken—and he loved chocolate and Coke.

Dr. Joseph took him off his much-loved chocolate and Coke,
primarily because of the caffeine, and added that he would like
for him to take vitamin C daily to boost his immune system.
The teacher thought the vitamin C that the boy was taking
every day was the Ritalin, and the mother allowed her to believe this. Dr. Joseph also began Alex on a treatment plan of
full spinal adjustments. Two weeks later, his mother reported
that things had improved greatly. She said the boy was much
calmer and more receptive to things around him, and he was-
n't fidgeting nearly as much as before. The teacher agreed that
the "drug" had done wonders for him.

Every child reacts to adjustments differently, of course, but it
is something every parent of learning disabled children should
consider. Trying a method that will not harm the child, and
will, in all probability, help him or her is not a very hard choice
to make.

## VACCINATIONS

For some parents, the decision of whether or not to vaccinate
their child is a very difficult one to make. We are all victims
of the daily pressure from the medical profession, society, government, school, and even the family to follow the path of least
resistance.

Many medical doctors *demand* that you vaccinate your child
or find another doctor. Parents are intimidated into believing
that if they don't get their child vaccinated, then they are
putting his or her health in great jeopardy. The government
claims you cannot go to school without immunization. The drug
companies use tremendously potent forms of advertising to try
to scare you into submission. Yet there are some strong, crys-
tal clear, and even frightening reasons *not* to vaccinate your
child. It is a choice *you* have to make.

J. Patrick writes in the article "The Great American Decep-
tion," as printed in the December 1976 issue of *Let's Live*,
"Vaccines are killing children. There is no doubt about it. We've
got figures to show it. It's damaging them, and in the United

Kingdom there is now a society for parents of vaccine-damaged children."

I will continue to repeat that the immune system is still the body's most effective weapon in the battle to protect and heal itself. The anti-vaccine movement is not only supported by the chiropractic community and other alternative health-care professionals but by a growing number of medical professionals as well. "The greatest threat of childhood disease lies in the dangerous and ineffectual efforts made to prevent them through mass immunization," said pediatrician Robert Mendelsohn, M.D. "Much of what you have been led to believe about immunizations simply isn't true. I not only have grave misgivings about them; if I were to follow my deep convictions . . . I would urge you to reject all inoculations for your child."

## There She Is . . . Miss America

Heather Whitestone, the former Miss America, is a good example of the way the public is sometimes misled by the media or of what is fed to the media, which, in turn, feeds us. Her deafness gave us a perfect example of the harm vaccinations can do, but the truth was covered up because the drug companies did not want parents to become frightened (or enlightened) about getting DPT shots for their children.

Heather Whitestone, an extremely lovely and talented young woman, was voted Miss America in 1994. Much has been mentioned in the media about her being a positive role model for both disabled and able-bodied young people. The 21-year-old Alabaman overcame the limitations of her profound deafness to become the first disabled contestant ever to win the Miss America contest, winning some $37,000 in scholarships and a personal appearance package worth more than $250,000.

Do you know what caused Ms. Whitestone's deafness?

Her mother, Daphne Gray, who obviously had not been coached initially by the Miss America Pageant's public relations department, first told reporters that her daughter was perfectly healthy until she received her DPT shot and that this shot was responsible for her deafness. The following day, the American Academy of Pediatrics reported in *The Washington Post* that "parents might be scared away from immunizing their children."

In the days that followed, several stories appeared about "what happened to Heather," yet none of them mentioned the DPT shot again. Later, other newspapers listed the cause of her deafness as a high fever. Mrs. Gray had already told the national television audience as well as the newspapers that it was the shot that was responsible—not a bacterial infection, the excuse that was later given—for Heather's deafness. Later, Mrs. Gray was quoted as saying her 18-month-old child had lost her hearing as a side effect of drugs that saved her life.

This devoted mother must have been advised that the truth might hurt other children whose parents would be afraid to get them vaccinated, and, as a result, her statements were adjusted to accommodate the public relations factor.

Can we not be trusted with the *truth* so that we can make our own decisions? Can we hear that Miss America's deafness was caused by her DPT shot and decide for ourselves whether we want to risk our children's health by having them receive the shot, or to refrain? Are we so stupid that we cannot make intelligent decisions for ourselves and our children? Do we have to be protected by those who think they know better? Who knows better than whom?

## Other Vaccination Dangers

I do not believe that the much lesser danger of the child contracting the disease is outweighed by the danger of the vaccines themselves. Doctors don't always report reactions, and those that are reported are sometimes the result of some special study commissioned by the government or the American Medical Association. A recent University of California—Los Angeles (UCLA) study estimates that as many as one in every thirteen children had persistent high-pitched crying after the DPT shot. Now, their crying may not necessarily be the result of the pain of the actual injection. According to Bobby Young, M.D., this may be indicative of brain damage in the recipient child. "The probability of causing damage is the same each time," Dr. Young said. "My greatest fear is that very few of them escape some kind of neurological damage out of this."

Many parents aren't aware that most infectious diseases began to decline long before the advent of vaccinations. According to the World Health Organization there has been a steady decline of infectious diseases in most developing countries. It appears that generally improved conditions of sanitation are largely responsible for the prevention of infectious disease. There are actual statistics and records from around the world that show that infectious diseases such as whooping cough, scarlet fever, and smallpox began to disappear long before immunizations came on the scene.

Even the dreaded polio's occurrences run in cycles. Without the vaccine, polio came and went in the first and third decades of this century. After it had peaked in 1949 and was subsiding naturally, it picked up again in 1952 when mass vaccination began. When it began to fall off again, the Salk vaccine was given the credit. Parents whose daily fears of the dreaded polio had held them captive were happy to believe there was something to stop this terrible threat. Although it is commonly believed that the Salk vaccine halted the polio epidemics that plagued American children in the 1940s and 1950s, why did the disease end in Europe as well, where the polio vaccine was not used nearly as much? Furthermore, 40 percent of our population was not immunized against polio. So where did it go, and why didn't it still attack those who were unprotected? I would imagine you will ask yourself this as well.

C. Kent, in the January 1983 issue of *Health Freedom News*, wrote an article entitled "Drugs, Bugs and Shots" in which he presented some information that is difficult for many to digest. "Statistics were 'cooked' to prove that the mass inoculation campaign was working. Cases formerly reported as polio were now reported as meningitis. So while polio statistics dropped, statistics for viral or aseptic meningitis soared."

Our government sometimes seems as confused as the general public about the whole business of vaccines. In 1984, the organization Health, Education, and Welfare (H.E.W.) reported that as many as 26 percent of children receiving a rubella vaccination in national testing programs developed arthralgia and arthritis, and some were hospitalized to be tested for rheumatic fever and rheumatic arthritis. The Assistant Secretary of Health in 1985, Edward Brandt, Jr., M.D., reported that every year, 35,000 children suffered neurological reactions because of the DPT shot.

According to Paavo Airola, a journalist who began researching adverse reactions to immunizations after noticing a prevail-
ing problem, "Two years ago [1977], we started to collect details from parents [regarding] serious reactions suffered by their
children to immunizations of all kinds. In 65 percent of the
cases referred to us, reactions followed 'triple' vaccinations. The
children in this group total 182 to date [1979]; all are severely
brain damaged, some are also paralyzed, and five have died
during the past 18 months. . . . Is it any wonder that some
doctors have called vaccinations 'legalized child abuse'?" she
said.

If none of this bothers you, consider some of the sources
from which these baby vaccines are made. Some vaccines are
made up of pig or horse blood, cowpox pus, rabbit brain tissue, dog kidney tissue, and duck egg protein. The polio vaccine contains a monkey kidney cell culture and calf serum. The
MMR (measles, mumps, and rubella) vaccine includes chick em-
bryos, and the DPT vaccine contains formaldehyde (used in em-
balming corpses) and aluminum phosphate (used in antiperspi-
rants as a drying agent.) C. Horowitz, writing in the journal
*Mothering* noted that most parents who feed their children properly would not let them eat food that contained any of the ingredients of immunization formulas.

As far back as 1937, W. H. Hay made the ineffectiveness of
vaccines evident in the *Congressional Record*. "It's nonsense to
think you can inject pus . . . into a little child and in any way
improve its health. . . . The body has its own methods of defense. These depend on the vitality of the body at the time. If
it is vital enough. it will resist all infections: if it isn't vital
enough, it won't, and you can't change the vitality of the body
for the better by introducing poison of any kind into it."

Consider these materials listed by the British National Anti-
Vaccination League as being used in vaccines:

Materials from which vaccines and serums are produced: rotten horse blood for diphtheria toxin and antitoxin; pulverized
felt hats for tetanus serum; sweepings from vacuum cleaners
for asthma and hayfever serums; pus from sores on diseased
cows for smallpox serums; mucous from the throats of children with colds and whooping cough for whooping cough

serum; decomposed fecal matter from typhoid patients for typhoid serum.

*The Physician's Desk Reference (PDR)*, the medical doctor's own manual for prescribing medication, states:

Injections of foreign substances—viruses, toxins, and foreign proteins—into the bloodstream, i.e. vaccinations, have been associated with diseases and disorders of the blood, brain, nervous system, and skin. Rare diseases such as atypical measles and monkey fever, as well as well-known disorders as premature aging and allergies have been associated with vaccinations.

Another thing that should concern us as parents is the safety of the vaccines themselves. Even if the ingredients of vaccines did not harm the children, some of what is referred to as "bad batches" have been causing any number of problems. Bad batches are specific lots of a vaccine that seem to cause an inordinate number of problems, adverse reactions, and deaths.

Kristine Severyn, a registered pharmacist with a doctoral degree in biopharmaceuticals and director of Ohio Parents for Vaccine Safety, expressed a grave concern that she shares with many parents about the safety of vaccines in a June 1994 guest editorial in the *Akron Beacon Journal*. In this article, she cites examples of the Food and Drug Administration's ineffectiveness in ensuring the safety and effectiveness of vaccines for children in this country. "For example, within a 39-month period ending November, 1993, the FDA's Vaccine Adverse Events Reporting System (VAERS) collected nearly 32,000 reports of bad reactions following vaccinations, with more than 700 deaths."

She writes that while the FDA acknowledges that this figure probably underestimates the actual number of adverse reactions due to the voluntary reporting system, little is done about it. "Instead of taking these reports of death and injury seriously, the FDA dismisses them as coincidental, so the reports languish in a government computer data base. This violates the intent of Congress when it established VAERS in the National Childhood Vaccine Act of 1986, as well as the FDA's statutory obligation to assure safe and effective vaccines."

Dr. Severyn goes on to point out in the article that when motivated, the FDA and medical communities can act decisively. She cites the FDA's embargo on improperly labeled orange juice and the American Medical Association's recommended ban on baby walkers, following the deaths of six children over a period of three years. She also mentioned the NBC news program *NOW*, where it was reported that one family discovered, through the Freedom of Information Act, that the lot of the DPT vaccine that permanently brain-damaged their child was already known by the FDA to be connected to six previous deaths. The lot continued to be used and at the time of the NBC broadcast, the FDA had received further reports of ten deaths from that same lot. Do you think the love of money could be involved here? I do.

The ten deaths were still considered *insufficient evidence* to cause them to withdraw the vaccine from use. The parents of these dead children would consider this a travesty. This is extremely frightening to parents and those concerned about the health of children in our country.

"The Ohio Department of Health also appears unconcerned about vaccine safety," Dr. Severyn continues. She reported that in eleven of twelve lots of DPT vaccine recently purchased by the Ohio Department of Health (ODH), significant numbers of adverse reaction reports had been received by the federal government, including twenty-seven deaths as of October 31, 1993. ODH was formally notified of this situation but failed to respond.

Dr. Severyn also discusses the inefficacy of the pertussis, or whooping cough, vaccine. She wrote that between 1987 and 1991, one-half of the reported cases of whooping cough, where vaccinated status was known, occurred in vaccinated children, according to Ohio's health department. Similarly, in 1993, the Chicago Department of Health noted that of 186 confirmed cases of pertussis, 72 percent of the children were up to date with their immunizations.

Dr. Severyn cites action against these ineffective vaccines taken in other countries. Germany has withdrawn the routine use of the pertussis vaccine, and Sweden discontinued its use years ago, due to poor efficacy and high incidence of adverse reactions. Both countries have had virtually no problems with whooping cough since then.

Toward the end of her article, Dr. Severyn adds that the current ambivalence of the FDA toward adverse vaccine reaction reports has caused parents to lose faith in our country's vaccination program. "Is it any wonder," she writes, "that some families refuse to expose their children to products that the FDA licenses then proceeds to forget?"

Dr. Severyn concluded with the following: "The public is repeatedly told that the benefits of vaccine outweigh the risks. Yet, we do not know what the risks are because our government is not interested, or perhaps afraid to find out. It's time for the FDA to do its job of properly monitoring safety and efficacy of licensed vaccines."

These are just some of the reasons why chiropractors feel strongly against the use of vaccinations and medical drugs. It's a money thing, I believe. I believe a life is more important than the pharmaceutical companies making more money. Don't you?

## Adults Need to Beware as Well

To continue with facts that some will call scare tactics, I would like to recount a recent news story. The Senate Committee of Veterans Affairs, headed by Senator Jay Rockefeller of West Virginia, announced in a fifty-three-page report that vaccines given to U.S. troops during the Persian Gulf War to protect them from chemical or biological weapons may be the cause of the mysterious illness collectively labeled "Gulf War Syndrome." The Pentagon did not get consent from many of those soldiers given the drug because of a wartime waiver granted by the Food and Drug Administration. However, officials were required to warn everyone of the risk of the drugs. This was not done, according to the report. They also pointed out that some of the soldiers were threatened with punishment if they did not obey orders to take the chemicals. In addition, they were also ordered to tell no one about their vaccinations, the report said. The report and its findings are still being studied.

Unfortunately, it was also noted that the drugs used to make the vaccine, pyridostigmine and botulinum toxin, most likely *would not* have protected the troops against possible chemical or biological weapons if they had been used by the Iraqi forces during the war.

I have never been *totally* opposed to the use of drugs and medical help under certain circumstances because there are times when some drugs are necessary for a patient's well being, and even to save his or her life. What I'm trying to make very clear is my wish to prevent patients from reaching that point in their lives where it will be necessary for them to resort to these methods. These methods should be at the bottom of the list—used only as a very last resort.

In a study conducted in the Spring of 1989 and recorded in the *Journal of Chiropractic Research*, it was found that sixty-three unvaccinated children between the ages of 8 and 15 who had been under chiropractic care had "increased resistance to the common childhood diseases—specifically measles, mumps, German measles, and chicken pox." This is what I am striving for—natural immunity.

Chiropractors have traditionally opposed immunization and instead promote natural health care, including natural childbirth, a good diet, breastfeeding, regular exercise, spinal checkups, and avoidance of drugs and surgery. We believe this will do more for a child's—or anyone's—natural immunity than any injections of artificial chemical additions. We also have the healthy children to back up this claim.

What I've found in my fifteen years of practice is that if you take your baby to a chiropractor, your friends will notice that your child is not getting sick all the time like the other kids. It happens to me as a parent, and my patients tell me it happens to them. Some of the parents may ask questions. When you tell them that your children are receiving regular chiropractic care, they often stare at you in disbelief. They did not get the answer they expected, and many are so narrow-minded (and medically conditioned) that they will not consider the health benefits of any type of alternative health care. For the most part, they will continue to give their sick children drugs, and you'll probably end up giving them a copy of this book in the sincere hope that they will give further consideration to the overall health benefits chiropractic can offer their children—and them as well. You've heard the old saying "You can lead a horse to water, but you can't make him drink," haven't you? Well, that's true, but if you want him to eat his oats, you can salt them. That's what I'm trying to do—salt people's oats with the truth.

Chiropractic adjustments are important to people of *all* ages. And since our children are treasured beyond measure, shouldn't we include them in our good-health-care plans? Periodic checkups will give your child the best opportunity possible to become not only the smartest kid in the class, but more important, the healthiest—and most likely—the happiest kid in the class.

And you won't have to tell your child. Like the boy on Art Linkletter's show—he'll notice it himself!

# Chapter 10

# Untarnishing the Golden Years

*Roger had just returned from his 40th class reunion and was discussing his trip with a couple of his friends.*

*"Well, did you have a good time?" one asked.*

*"Oh sure," Roger answered. "It was great."*

*"How did everybody look?" another inquired.*

*"Oh, they all looked pretty good," Roger replied. "Except some of them were so fat, bald, and old-looking, that they didn't even recognize me."*

Age, of course, is just a simple case of mind over matter, as some have said. If you don't *mind*, it doesn't *matter*. Regardless of what we claim, we all worry about getting older. But if we think of the alternative, we realize that our choices are rather limited. Perhaps we should worry about *not* getting older. What we should be concerned about is getting older *without* getting sick. Most people think of "old" and "sick" in the same breath, when they should be thinking "older and healthier." To reach our so-called golden years only to find pain and distress is certainly nothing to look forward to. But to sail into what could be the best years of our lives feeling great and enjoying life to the fullest is something worthy of our most desired goals. It makes a well-funded 401K plan look paltry.

I believe the older we get, the more *productive* we should be;

the older we get, the *wiser* we ought to be; the older we get, the more *respected* we ought to be; even more important, the older we get, the *healthier* we ought to be.

As we age, the "golden years" should indeed be golden—happy, less stressed, and relaxed, yet active. Your children are grown and gone. The house is paid off. You have retired from the daily grind, and it's time to reap the benefits you've worked toward all your life. It's time to volunteer with your favorite charity, to travel, to read the books you've put off reading, to take walks in the park, to take up painting, to try skydiving, and to completely enjoy yourself and your surroundings. It's time you did what you've always wanted to do.

What's wrong with this picture? What is reality? It's not quite as rosy as it should be. Too many older people are no longer pillars in their communities. Some step down from being chairperson of the board to become simply bored out of their chair. Some become like ghosts. We see them, but we actually look right through them because we fail to see what an important role they can play in our day-to-day lives. We fail to give them the attention they deserve. It is painful today to take note of how little respect some of our young people give their elders. Their opinions are neither sought nor valued. Their years of experience and wisdom are often belittled as being "old-fashioned" or "out of step with the times." After all, this is the nineties. Get with it.

Add to all of this the fact that many older people simply don't feel well. They are, in fact, miserable and see no other future but more misery and monthly (sometimes weekly) trips to the doctor's office just to get another bottle of pills to add to their already overflowing medicine cabinet. They are not living a life. They are simply seeking relief from pain that keeps them from living.

An even sadder commentary is the reaction of some of the older people to their "place in life."

"Well, that's the way it is when you get old . . ."

"Can't expect to be in good health after all these years."

"I've had a pretty good life . . ."

They seem to accept this terrible fate and in many cases prefer not to be involved in the lives of younger people at all. It's simply too difficult to put forth the effort. It's easier to say,

"Well, the young folks these days are different from the way we were when we were young." There is also a certain "grumpy old man or woman" attitude of, "Hey, leave me alone. I've done my share of work. Find your own answers, the way I did."

Older age does not mean you should be relegated to the back of the line—shoved out of the way, so to speak—in deference to those movers and shakers who are young, vital, and "getting things done." Because of your age and experience, you should be sought for answers. People should come to you for advice. Your opinions or your advice does not have to be followed to the letter, but it should be valued and considered worthwhile. *If you learn to place a greater value on yourself, people will naturally think you are of greater value.* We are all of *great value,* otherwise we would never have been created in the first place!

## AGE IS ONLY A THREE-LETTER WORD

It saddens me to say that one of the reasons (maybe the biggest reason) more older people do not become involved in the lives of others, the reason they wither away in a corner somewhere and ask to be left alone is that they just do not feel well. Their health does not permit them to enjoy life or to share it with anyone else. A person has to feel good about him- or herself before he or she can help anyone else. And in order to feel good about him- or herself, he or she first has to *feel good!*

Too many older adults look, act, think, and feel *old.* As a result, they *are* old—sometimes as early as in their forties. They have become old simply because they do not feel well. What a shame. That's not the way it has to be. I do not believe it is our Creator's plan for anyone to be sickly and die at an early age, often filled with bitterness, anxiety, and pain. I do not believe God would have a baby brought into the world who is going to "fall apart" by the age of fifty or sixty. I don't accept growing older as a diagnosis for sickness.

I hear it in my office all the time. In fact, I hear it everywhere I go. People will say things like, "Oh, I'm just *getting old.* . . . Gotta expect all these aches and pains at my age." Not on your healthy life, you don't. I believe the bodies we live in have the ability to maintain good health many more years than what is now acknowledged. It's not our bodies that betray us; it is the *manner* in which we treat our bodies that causes them to give out.

I know we're all going to die someday. But my point is wouldn't it be better if we died from just plain being worn out after a very long and healthy life? I've discussed this a lot in this book, but I cannot stress enough the importance of *quality* of life along with the *quantity*. I don't believe one has to be sacrificed for the other. You and I both know it would be much better to reach the age of 95, and, after having worked in your garden all day, lie down in your own bed for sleep and die peacefully. Unfortunately, it is much more common to hear of one dying at the age of 66, 70, or 73 after suffering with arthritis for twenty years, developing diabetes and high blood pressure, and not really enjoying those golden years at all—just getting by. This cannot be called living. It is only *existing*. There *is* a better way. There is the way that I believe our Creator planned for us. He wanted us to live a long, healthy, fruitful, sharing, giving life. Doesn't that make sense to you?

## A BETTER WAY

I am a strong believer in the concept of one thinking for one's self, and that may sound funny coming from someone who has written an entire book giving you insights on what to think. Remember, though, I am not telling you *what* to think, I am offering you alternatives to the mainstream ideas of maintaining your good health. We must be educated about real health, not educated about sickness. We must seek answers to the age-old question of not only how to live long, but also how to live well.

What do we need to *do* in order to become and remain healthy? There are some very basic answers here, yet one of the biggest problems I've seen is the inability to control the all-important "self." Self-discipline is probably the hardest aspect of controlling our health problems. I think that most of us, deep down inside our hearts, know of many things in our lives that we could change in order to help us enjoy a healthier life, yet we do not listen to this inner voice. We'd rather do what we want to do, and hope we can be well without having to do any additional work. We know we should exercise, but we tell ourselves that we do not have the time. We try to eat right but decide it is too expensive, is too difficult, or simply does not taste good.

Magazines, newspapers, and television screens are filled with advertisements that try to tell us how to "correct" our health problems. There is no talk of how you came to suffer from all these ailments in the first place, or even how to heal them permanently; these ads only discuss how to put the pain away as quickly as possible. There are endless confusing and contradicting statements coming from the medical profession. One doctor says jog; one says not to. One says vitamins are good; One says vitamins are bad. One study says some substance will harm you; another says it won't. When faced with all these "facts," we simply throw up our hands and say, "To heck with it all," and do as we please—which is not usually in our health's best interest.

I believe that some of that confusion is intended. If we all throw caution to the wind and stop worrying about what is good or bad for us, we will most likely err on the side of ill health. And if we get sick, we'll go to the doctor, get medicine to mask the pain, and go on with our lives as usual.

Is this the answer? You know it's not. We need to be thoroughly educated about what is right and what is wrong for our bodies. That, too, takes a lot of time and effort that we neither have nor want to expend. We need to learn how to take care of ourselves—and *do it!*

It is sad to say, but sickness is a big business. The more people who are sick, the more money is made by the medical industry. Trillions of dollars are made annually in the "sickness business." Unfortunately, there is not nearly as much to be made in the "good health" business.

It is extremely painful for me to walk through a nursing home and see the loss of hope, the helplessness, and the utter despair on the faces of many of the people. It is even more painful when I know there is *a better way,* and that they don't have to be warehoused in this manner. Their health could be improved. Their illnesses could be prevented. The health-care industry could be changed. We can get well. We can heal. And we can be happy. It isn't easy, and it takes time and effort. You've heard the old saying that accomplishing anything worthwhile takes effort. Well, what could be more worthwhile than working toward your good health? We spend a lifetime studying to upgrade our career, to select the right kind of financial portfolio, to build an impressive estate—and for what? If you are not healthy, none of these things will be worth a hill of organically grown beans to you. Your unhealthy heirs will probably waste it all anyway. We are well aware that people's attitudes and ingrained training cannot be changed overnight, but there has to be a change in the way things are being done today.

Wouldn't it be wonderful if we could close all the nursing homes? I'm not saying that's possible. There is a certain (albeit limited) need for these types of facilities in today's world. There are many—far too many—sick older people who cannot do for themselves, have no one who can care for them, and are likely never to be any better. They did not plan ahead for a healthy old age, so they need help and care, and we must give it to them. The giving souls working and volunteering in many nursing homes, offering loving care to these people are to be highly commended; just as those who neglect them are to be condemned. As the average age of our society increases, it becomes more and more apparent that housing the elderly in nursing homes is not the best way of dealing with our older citizens.

Why is this happening? Is it that we don't love our parents and grandparents? Have we become unfeeling and uncaring as well as disrespectful to our elders? Before answering these questions, let us set the record straight now. I know there are some cases in which it is absolutely necessary for an older person to be placed in a clean, well-staffed, well-equipped, caring nursing facility (which is the condition of many nursing homes). Unfortunately, there are too many of the "other" kind, which are simply dirty warehouses charging a king's ransom to house, medicate, and neglect your loved ones until they die.

The fact that our current generation of senior citizens is the first senior generation to, for the most part, live alone, outside the bonds of an extended family does not say much for our society today. This is also the first generation of senior citizens to be extensively medicated, often by several doctors who do not tell each other what they have prescribed. Our elderly are not only excessively drugged and malnourished, they are often severely depressed and alone, waiting for the one event they see as postive—death.

There are other alternatives. I cannot stress enough the importance of searching for and finding ways of maintaining your health while you are young. However, if you did not do this, all is not lost—there are still many ways you can help restore your health, no matter what age you are. I'm sure you've heard the comedian who said if he had known he was going to live so long, he would have taken better care of himself. There is a lot of truth in that statement.

The boundaries of old age are being redefined. There are many scientists who believe that life does not have to end at 85, or 100, or even 120. Others (usually those far younger) shrink back in horror at this suggestion. The population is too great now, they say, and what we need is less people, not (old) people who live on and on. Do you find these statements as frightening as I do?

Who will decide how long we live? It's hard for some of us to believe that several years ago, there was the idea in the younger generation (and a movie based on this idea, I believe) that everyone *over thirty years of age* should be "put to sleep." Of course, most of those making that suggestion were amazed to discover that when they reached the age of thirty, (rapidly, I might add) this no longer seemed like a good idea.

Do you think someone should be in charge of the time we are destined to die? In whose hands do you want that decision to lie? A blue-ribbon panel of judges? Your doctor? Your family? Your church? A committee? Most of us, if we feel reasonably well, do not wish to hasten that final exit, regardless of what is written and taught about the "dignity of dying." I'd much rather talk about the "dignity of living well."

## STAYING HEALTHY LATER IN LIFE

Statistics now tell us that Americans are living longer and healthier lives. In 1970, the number of those known to have reached the age of 100 or older was less than 3,000. By 1980, the number had jumped to more than 14,000. Are these older

Americans well? Is the quality of their lives worth living that long? Those are questions that could only be answered by those who have reached that milestone.

You may be surprised to find that old age does not have to mean being sick. Studies have shown that it is possible to live a long, full life without being physically or mentally incapacitated. You may have great difficulty visualizing this, but try getting a sharp image of one of the health spas we have today (usually overflowing with the young and beautiful) filled to capacity with groups of 60-, 70-, and even 80-year-olds, all working out on the weight machines. Well, if you're young, you're probably laughing, and even if you're older, you may still be laughing. But listen, exercise is not only for the young. It is *definitely* for the elderly as well. Exercise maven Bonnie Prudden has been quoted as saying, "While you can't turn back the clock . . . you can wind it up again."

In a pilot study conducted by Dr. Marie Fiatarone of Tufts University and Harvard Medical School, nine people from 86 to 90 years of age worked out using a weight machine three times a week. They increased the strength of their quadriceps by an average of 174 percent. One of the participants, 92-year-old Dorothy Tishler, related that she thought they were "cuckoo" when they first asked her if she wanted to "pump some iron." Later, she admitted that she had been a fool to doubt the effect. "They made a new person out of me," she said.

Most older people have accepted "the fact" that they will fall into severe mental decline and suffer from senility, which they have been programmed to believe is inevitable. Repeat after me. *Sickness and loss of intelligence is not a normal aging process.* It's true that we won't be as agile or as alert as we once were, but studies have proven that age problems may consist mostly of ideas of aging that have been implanted in the mind. As I said in the beginning of this chapter—it's mind over matter.

In his book *Quantum Healing*, best-selling author and lecturer Deepak Chopra writes:

> Careful study of healthy elderly people—as opposed to the sick, hospitalized ones whom medicine habitually studies—has revealed that 80 percent of healthy Americans, barring psychological distress (such as loneliness, depression, or lack of

outside stimulation), suffer no significant memory loss as they age. As long as a person stays mentally active, he/she will remain as intelligent as in youth and middle age.

I think this is extremely encouraging, but how often do you read statements such as this? Most of the time we accept the fact that the older you are, the less able you are to do (or remember) anything.

Negativity is another tool used to control. People who feel good about themselves have a healthy outlook on life, are positive people, and are in control of themselves. A person who is positive and upbeat is not an easy target for those who wish to control their thoughts.

## CHIROPRACTIC AND ALZHEIMER'S DISEASE

Alzheimer's disease is a terrible degenerative disease of the brain that can cause confusion; memory loss; delirium; restlessness; and problems with perception, speech, and locomotion. It was first identified in a 51-year-old patient by a German physician named Alois Alzheimer in 1906. Since this time, research done by the standard medical profession has cast very little light on the cause of this extremely debilitating condition. So far, we are told that this mysterious and irreversible death of the mind cannot be prevented, treated, or cured. Although it can occur in younger people, more than two-thirds of the victims of Alzheimer's disease are 65 or older, with 25 percent of Alzheimer's disease patients over the age of 85.

Alzheimer's disease is not easy to diagnose, since it shares symptoms with various other ailments such as anemia, thyroid disease, vitamin deficiency, mini-strokes, depression, and even alcoholism. Furthermore, several classes of drugs used in the fight against asthma, Parkinson's disease, hypertension, and depression can also cause symptoms much like those of Alzheimer's disease. According to the 1989 *Drug Interactions and Side Effects Index* to the *Physician's Desk Reference*, there are twenty-eight drugs that can cause memory impairment, fourteen drugs that can cause short-term memory loss, six drugs that can cause dementia, and twenty-one that can cause delusions. All of these effects are also symptoms of Alzheimer's disease.

The prognosis for an Alzheimer's disease patient is extremely depressing. Eventually, the victim loses all control over bodily functions, and his or her ultimate descent into a coma is followed by death. The average course of the disease is eight years, but it can last as little as three, or as long as twenty-five years. Similar brain tissue deterioration and reduced levels of certain brain chemicals are revealed in the autopsies of most of the victims.

There are some new clues to the cause of Alzheimer's disease, but the jury is still out on the exact cause, prevention, and/or cure. Some researchers believe that spinal structural imbalance can be a partial cause of the disease. According to Dr. Lowell Ward, D.C., spinal imbalance puts pressure on the spinal cord and can squeeze and severely damage the lower brain or brain stem and affect the function of the brain. Dr. Ward is one of the few lights at the end of the dark tunnel, reporting several cases of Alzheimer's disease reversal with chiropractic treatment.

An interesting article on the subject appeared in the April 1986 edition of *The New England Journal of Medicine.* It discussed studies showing that in 10 to 20 percent of cases of Alzheimer's disease, the patient had suffered serious head injuries up to thirty-five years prior to the onset of the disease. This would lead me to believe that old injuries to the head and/or neck could play some part in the cause of this ailment.

As an alternative health-care method, chiropractic care is certainly something to be considered for overall good health—including the prevention of Alzheimer's disease. Since spinal imbalance seems to play a role in the development of Alzheimer's disease, it is important to have regular spinal adjustments as a preventative measure against the disease. Chiropractic has also been found to have some effect on the reversal of Alzheimer's disease. I believe chiropractic care is important, not only for those already suffering from Alzheimer's disease, but for those who are serious about their general well-being. In light of standard medicine's failure to offer any solutions to the problem of Alzheimer's disease, I believe we need to look further into all alternative methods of health care such as chiropractors, nutritionists, homeopaths, exercise physiologists, acupuncturists, and practitioners of various other body work disciplines.

## CHIROPRACTIC AND OSTEOPOROSIS

Osteoporosis is a disorder characterized by degeneration of the bone. This condition that often causes pain, frequent broken bones, loss of height, and malformation of body parts usually affects postmenopausal women and inactive, often elderly, patients. I don't think we are doomed to suffer from osteoporosis or any other illness. I think we were meant to use our God-given common sense to take care of ourselves. While it is true that osteoporosis is quite prevalent in older patients, it does not have to be an accepted fact of life.

According to researcher J. Lee in "Osteoporosis Reversal, The Role of Progesterone," which appeared in the July 1990 issue of *The International Clinical Nutrition Review* "True reversal of osteoporosis has [been proven] unobtainable by conventional methods."

Most of us are aware of the pros and cons of estrogen replacement therapy. Utilizing small doses of estrogen can be effective in slowing the rate of bone breakdown, but it carries the serious long-term risk of increased exposure to certain cancers.

I cannot stress how important it is for older patients to take full advantage of chiropractic care. It has been proven helpful for the elderly, especially those who suffer from diseases of aging such as osteoporosis or Alzheimer's disease. Chiropractic care relieves the body of spinal nerve stress and can help improve a person's chance of healing him- or herself naturally. Osteoporosis sufferers can benefit greatly from chiropractic care. Those who are not osteoporosis victims (or are unaware of it) could save themselves a lot of pain and disabilities by taking advantage of this alternative prevention and health-care method.

## JUST SAY NO!!!

What do you think of when you hear the "Just Say No" slogan? Young people in the midst of a drug culture? While that image is certainly often appropriate, there is a lot more to consider when it comes to drugs. It might surprise you to learn that the most "drugged-up" group in American culture today is not the "reckless youth," but our older Americans. The sever-

# *Did You Know...*

... that regular weight-bearing activity has been shown to increase or maintain bone density, an important step in the prevention of osteoporsis?

ity of the senior ctizen drug problem would put the problem of all other categories of drug abusers to shame. We are overrun by this serious and still-growing problem.

The elderly account for 51 percent of all deaths from drug reactions. In 1987 alone, an estimated 200,000 senior citizens entered hospitals due to adverse drug reactions or overdoses. There are more than 2 million elderly addicted, or at the risk of being addicted, to minor tranquilizers or sleeping pills. And every year 63,000 senior citizens experience serious mental impairment either caused or worsened by the taking of drugs. An even sadder thought may be that these statistics are just the tip of the iceberg.

Just say no . . . *to your medical doctor.*

Oh, I can't do that, you say. My doctor will get mad and won't give me any more magic bullets. If your medical doctor is concerned at all about you and your total well-being, he or she will listen to your fears about the overuse of drugs and will help you break, or at least lessen, your drug habit. If your doctor does not at least consider your fears and concerns, then you must realize you have a doctor whose priorities are directed toward his or her bankbook and not your health chart. Look for a new doctor. Older Americans are the prime victims of doctor abuse. They ingest too many drugs and are subjected to other forms of medical intervention that rob them of their health, their decision-making freedom, and, all too often, their very lives.

Older Americans seldom sneak down to the corner and buy their drugs from some slimy-looking guy driving a fancy car. They walk into the drug store with a permit from their doctors and purchase them legally. Legal use does not, however, make it safe. In 1989, the United States Government issued a report in which Richard P. Kusserow, Inspector General of the

Department of Health and Human Services, said that the improper use of drugs, misdiagnoses by doctors, and inappropriate dosage levels are "widespread problems" among the elderly. Is there such a thing as elder abuse? Of course there is.

Just because you have entered the so-called golden years does not mean you are immediately rendered senseless. The elderly have a responsibility to take care of themselves and to take charge of their own good health—as we all should be doing all our lives. It's your life. Granted, the medical industry turns some individuals into passive recipients of impersonal procedures and overdrugged victims of a medical run-around that too often refuses (or fails to understand) the holistic health benefits of nutrition, exercise, and other nonmedical alternatives. The bottom line is that the older patient has to learn to watch out for him- or herself. Unfortunately, many of the elderly accept the "good doctor's" word for everything, and they ignore the need for a well-rounded health-care regimen.

*"But I'm old,"* you may say. That's all the more reason you should listen! If nothing else, older Americans should pay particular attention to a recent study as reported in *The New York Times*. The headline alone should make you sit up and take notice: "Unnecessary Drugs Plague the Elderly." A study was conducted by Dr. Steffi Woolhandler, M.D., of Harvard Medical School and colleagues. They examined data from a national survey that included more than 6,000 older people who were not in nursing homes to find out what medicines they were taking.

They determined that close to a quarter of all Americans 65 or older had been given prescriptions for drugs that can produce such serious side effects as heart problems or respiratory failure. Even more frightening was the finding that some of the drugs also caused amnesia and confusion—symptoms of Alzheimer's disease (further proof that people may be diagnosed as having Alzheimer's disease, when actually their symptoms may be due to the effects of their medication). It was the conclusion of the investigators that it was unnecessary to prescribe these drugs to older people, either because safer alternatives are available or because the drugs "simply were not needed."

The researchers took a list of twenty drugs that a panel of experts said should not be prescribed for older people (see the inset on page 201), then compared the list with the drugs being taken by those in their study. They found, for example, that 1.8 million older people had prescriptions for dipyridamole, a blood thinner that researchers say is useless for all except those who have had artificial heart valves implanted. How many people had had this procedure at the time of this study? Only 36,000 Americans, half of them over 65, had heart valves implanted, yet almost 2 million were taking prescriptions that would only benefit those 36,000. Something is *very* wrong with a picture like that.

The researchers also found that more than 1.3 million older Americans had prescriptions for propoxyphene, an addictive narcotic that is no better than aspirin in relieving pain. More than 1.2 million were taking diazepam or chlordiazepoxide, long-acting sedatives that can not only make people groggy and forgetful, but can cause them to lose their balance as well resulting in dangerous falls. The authors of the study said they were actually conservative in their selection of the twenty drugs that should not be prescribed, meaning that there are actually several more drugs to be avoided.

Dr. Jerry H. Gurwitz, M.D. of Brigham and Women's Hospital in Boston wrote an editorial that accompanied the printing of the study in the *Times* stating that he hoped the study would serve as a "wake-up call" to America's doctors and added that he hoped the medical community would "take it as seriously as the general public, I think, will."

Dr. Gurwitz went further to say that he feared the study may have understated the problem, since it did not consider drug interactions or drugs such as sleeping pills that may be appropriate for a short time at a low dose but are often taken by older people for months or years, in dosages that can cause drowsiness and loss of memory.

"If a patient loses memory or loses balance," Dr. Gurwitz was quoted as saying, "they say it's old age."

This opinion was further echoed by Dr. Robert Butler, M.D., chairman of the Department of Geriatrics at Mount Sinai School of Medicine. It was also his opinion that it was not only the doctors who should bear the guilt of the misuse of drugs, but the older people themselves who shrug off the side effects of medication and attribute them to "the effects of old age" should also be held accountable.

# Drugs Considered Inappropriate for Older People

Following is a list of drugs that were determined by a Harvard study to be inappropriate for most of the elderly population as published in the *Journal of the American Medical Association*. The first name printed is the the drug's generic name. The names in parentheses following the generic name are the brand names under which the drug is sold. Each drug is followed by its detrimental effects. If you are elderly and any of these drugs have been prescribed for you, ask your doctor if he or she can prescribe an alternative medication. In some cases it may be necessary for some elderly patients to take one or some of these drugs for short periods of time, but long-term use of any of these drugs is ill-advised. This list, released in 1994, by no means includes all drugs inappropriate for the elderly.

*Tranquilizers and Sedatives:*

- Diazepam (Valium): Addictive and too long-acting, causing possible drowsiness, confusion, and falls.

- Chlordiazepoxide (Librium, Librax): Too long-acting, may cause falls.

- Flurazepam (Dalmane): Too long-acting, may cause falls.

- Meprobamate (Miltown, Deprol, Equagesic, Equanil). This drug is sometimes combined with an antidepressant or pain reliever: Addictive, too long-lasting, may cause falls.

- Pentobarbital (Nembutal): Addictive, long-acting.

- Secobarbital (Seconal): Addictive, long-acting.

*Antidepressants:*

- Amitriptyline (Elavil, Endep, Etrafon, Limbitrol, Triavil): Often causes dizziness, drowsiness, and inability to urinate in the elderly.

*Arthritis Drugs:*

- Indomethacin (Indocin): Can cause confusion and headaches. May be appropriate in some elderly patients under certain conditions.

- Phenylbutazone (Butazolidin): Risk of bone marrow toxicity.

*Diabetes Drugs:*

- Chlorpropramide (Diabinese): Can cause dangerous fluid retention and stays in the body a long time, so if an overdose occurs, it can take a long time to treat.

*Pain Relievers:*

- Propoxyphene (Darvon Compound, Darvocet, Wygesic): Addictive and little more effective than aspirin, has more side effects than morphine for patients who need a narcotic, and has been associated with seizures and heart problems.

- Pentazocine (Talwin): Addictive, has been associated with seizures and heart problems.

*Dementia Treatments:*

- Cyclandelate: Not shown to be effective.
- Isoxsuprine: Not shown to be effective.

*Blood Thinners:*

- Dipyridamole (Persantine): Except in patients with artificial heart valves, not shown to be effective.

*Muscle Relaxants:*

- Cyclobenzaprine (Flexeril): Can cause dizziness, drowsiness, and fainting.

- Orphenadrine (Norflex, Norgesic): Can cause dizziness, drowsiness, and fainting.

- Methocarbamol (Robaxin): May cause dizziness or drowsiness.

- Carisoprodol (Soma): Potential for central nervous system toxicity is greater than potential benefit.

*Antiemetics:*

- Trimethobenzamide (Tigan): May be less effective than other agents. May cause drowsiness, dizziness, and other adverse reactions.

*—From a Harvard Study in the Journal of the American Medical Association*

Dr. Butler said he often conducts what he calls a "brown bag test," where he asks his elderly patients to bring all their medication into his office in a bag. "You would be shocked," he said. "Sometimes Mrs. Jones next door got a good result with her arthritis medication, so our patient will take Mrs. Jones' drug. Some are taking medications that are five or six years old."

While I wholeheartedly agree with the basis and outcome of this impressive study, I do have difficulty with one very important fact. The survey was conducted in 1987, but the data was not made available for analysis until 1994. The researchers also indicated that there had been no similar studies conducted since that time. It took *seven* years from the time the study was completed to the time it was made available for the general public's information. What about all those people during that period of time who were unaware of the dangers? How many other things don't we know that we should know about? And, even more important, *why* was the information not made public right away, and *who* would want this vital information kept from the public?

It's very frightening.

Just as the study proved that there are ethical and caring medical doctors who are searching for and often finding answers to many of our health problems, there are those who are equally as anxious to keep those answers away from the people whose lives depend on that knowledge.

What it all comes down to is that the consumer must beware. Be educated and be careful about the kind of medication you put into your body. Age doesn't mean we have to accept what others say is right for us. We have not lost our minds just because we've had more birthdays. I subscribe to the late George Burns' philosophy, "You can't help getting older, but you don't have to get old." Well said, George! He lived to be 100, but he *never* got old.

I believe that far too many medical doctors use age as an excuse to get the person out of his or her office. They do not want to take the time or extend the effort and the energy it may require to determine what the patient really needs. So instead of doing a good examination, creating a thorough history, and engaging in meaningful dialogue with the patient, they simply dismiss his or her problems as "old age." They feel that the patient can't or won't get any better, so they write a prescription to get him or her out of the office to make room for the next patient. After all, these doctor are *very* busy. How many medical doctors do you know of who have enough time to sit and talk to you, to really inquire about your problems, and to actually study the situation and consider the best course of action?

"Here's a prescription, get it filled, and see if you feel better . . . if not, let me know, and I'll try something else."

Where does all this stop? It must stop with *you*. The doctor is *your* employee. *You* are paying for his or her services. What he or she says is not carved in stone anywhere. The doctor did not go up a mountain and bring down tablets that say you must be medicated. *You* are the one in charge, and you must not be intimidated into believing that *you* are not in control of *your* own good health. *You* must take responsibility for *your* own health and that of *your family*. Do not let the doctor control your common sense any longer. Seek *good* care from *good* doctors—doctors who understand *good* health. By this time you will not be surprised that chiropractors fit this description.

If I can end this chapter with one thought, it would be for you to read and reread what is written here. Read this book thoroughly and study its content. It will help to educate you about your own good health, and the more educated you become about your own good health, the healthier you will be.

And the healthier you are, the happier you'll be!

Read on . . .

# Chapter 11

# Exercise, Nutrition, and Good Old Common Sense

*Experience keeps a dear school,*
*but fools will learn in no other,*
*and scarcely in that;*
*for it is true,*
*we may give advice but we cannot give conduct.*
*Remember this;*
*they that will not be counseled*
*cannot be helped.*
*If you do not hear reason*
*she will rap you over your knuckles.*

—*Benjamin Franklin*

Take a walk! Eat your vegetables! Relax!

You've heard all this before. In fact, you've heard it so much that you no longer *hear* it at all. But I can assure you, it is still some of the best advice you will ever get. What I want you to do is wipe the slate clean, and let's begin again.

Take a walk . . . every day! Eat your vegetables, and make sure you have a well-balanced diet! Relax, and get rid of some of the stress in your life!

All right, I'm boring you . . . actually, I'm aggravating you. But this is *very important* and this time you are not only going to listen, but you are going to utilize this advice to maintain your good health for the rest of your (very long, I hope) life. I hope that sounded like a threat because that's the way it was meant.

What happens if you *don't* do as I say? Will I come after you, stalk you in restaurants, cut the strings on your hammock, and mail you cassettes of the seashore and soothing waterfall sounds? No, I won't do that, but I'll tell you what will happen. You could end up a sick old person.

This is serious business, folks, pay attention! Even if you are already past fifty or sixty or older, it's still not too late to follow a few simple rules, as you learned in Chapter 10. Hey, it's not gonna kill you if you follow them. I can't make that promise if you don't.

## EXERCISE

Usually when people talk or write about doing exercises, they follow their statements with, ". . . but before you begin any exercise or diet program, ask your doctor about it." Most people simply do not realize how little most medical doctors actually know about nutrition or exercise. Take a good look at our doctors. How many do you see who look like the perfect specimen of health? Not many. The same holds true for nurses. This is not a criticism nor is it meant to be cruel, but many of the people in our health-care system are grossly overweight, overstressed, and overworked. They are not models you'd want to emulate. Some weight-loss programs offer the warning about seeing your doctor first, of course, to help ward off lawsuits if something does go wrong in the program. They hope to have the medical doctor shoulder some of the blame—*if* the person did actually ask a doctor, which most people certainly don't.

The second reason you're told to see your doctor can be summed up in one word—*control*. It is part of the health-care system plan for controlling you. You can't possibly have any common sense of your own. *See your doctor.* Wouldn't it make even more sense to say, "before undertaking any exercise program, see your chiropractor"? Do you ever see or hear that? Of course you don't. We don't have that kind of control.

How many people ask their doctors about doing some type of moderate exercise such as walking, and the doctor responds, "No, I don't want you to exercise, and I don't want you to eat right either." Most people can exercise, even with many serious illnesses including diabetes, heart disease, high blood pressure, and arthritis as long as they understand the need for moderation. However, sometimes it is necessary to have a complete physical examination done to ensure that your body is in proper working order and that you have no limitations. This physical should include not only a medical examination, but a chiropractic examination as well.

As for asking your doctor about diet and nutrition, it's a good bet that if you are an avid or even a sometime reader, you probably know more than your doctor knows about what's good for you nutritionally. Now, before I am bombarded by letters from those doctors who *do* know something about nutrition—yes, I know you are out there. But you are certainly in the minority, and you know that as well as I do.

The exercises I'm talking about for the average person do not include massive body-building exercises or running in the Boston Marathon. I'm just talking about moving off the couch and allowing your body to operate the way it was designed to operate. One foot in front of the other. Easy does it.

How many people do you know of who suffered a heart attack after receiving a completely clean bill of health at their last checkup? Those of you who are old enough will remember that former President of the United States Dwight D. Eisenhower had a heart attack during his term as President, shortly after receiving a clean bill of health from his medical doctor. We all know that the former President had the best medical care he could possibly get, yet the doctor was still unable to predict this oncoming disaster. When you think of the more than half million people this year who will die from heart attacks, you cannot believe that you are so special that this illness will ignore you. You must *work* at being healthy. In the times in which we live today, with the pollution, toxic junk, and dangers that lurk in the air you breathe and the water you drink, we must, *at the very least*, give ourselves that little extra edge.

It's time to get moving, not after vacation, not next Monday, not the first day of next month, not January 1st, not even tomorrow. Today. Now. Move. You might want to finish this chapter first—then again you might want to come back to it after your walk.

You may ask yourself what is so important about being active? I think the best answer to that question is that motion is life, and the absence of motion is death. Can I get any plainer than that? The choice seems quite simple when put in those terms.

Exercise is a natural movement of the body. I believe that *any* exercise is better than *none*, and I'm also convinced that if you do not exercise, you won't be in good health for long. If you're not good to your body, it won't be good to you. It's that simple. Exercise helps oxygen and other nutrients get to all parts of the body, right down to the smallest cell. Exercise helps our bodies cleanse themselves and get rid of the toxins. By exercising, we cause the blood to move through the blood vessels of our whole body, strengthening, rebuilding, and repairing.

Except for those people who are unable to walk because of a physical disability, walking is considered to be the "universal exercise." Walking is just good common sense because you are using 200 muscles with every step you take. However, you must be careful not to overdo any activity, just as you should be careful not to park your behind on the couch and vegetate into oblivion. There are people who have become obsessive about exercise, and that's where common sense comes in. If you are one of those people who feel you must exercise vigorously every day of your life for hours at a time, you're probably overextending yourself. Unless you are in training for a television role as one of the *Baywatch* babes or hunks or, you are working out for the bathing suit issue of *Sports Illustrated*, you are overdoing it. Most of us have neither the time nor the inclination to spend this much time exercising. On the other hand, if you feel that a stroll to the refrigerator to get a bottle of beer constitutes your exercise for the day, you'll need to extend yourself a little bit more. I am still talking common sense here. What we have to do in all facets of our lives—and exercise is certainly no exception—is to find a balance that fits our own lifestyle and our own abilities.

# Did You Know...

. . . that research at the University of Southern California North Cancer Center involving more than 1,000 California women indicates as much as a 60-percent reduction in breast cancer among women who exercise regularly, particularly those who worked out for at least four hours a week?

. . . that studies into colon cancer at that same institute offer similar findings? According to Steven Blair, director of epidemiology at the Cooper Institute of Aerobics Research, men and women who participate in "higher levels" of leisure (tennis, anyone?) and occupational physical activity, experienced a significant reduction in colon cancer risk.

## How Do I Go About Getting Myself Motivated?

When I talk to my patients about exercising, I try to emphasize the obvious benefits such as an overall feeling of well-being. I tell them that exercise promotes better circulation and nerve function and greatly strengthens the immune system.

I also talk to my patients about a plan of action. Can you imagine any general ordering his or her troops into battle without a battle plan? It's a matter of life and death, and he or she wants to be sure of the outcome. It's the same with taking care of yourself. It's a matter of health and life, or death. We are in a fierce battle, people. Ask yourself how many times your conversation drifts to this ailment or that ailment when you are with a group of your friends. People are sick . . . and getting sicker.

I tell my patients they need to establish their plans of action and set their goals for a one-year period, month by month. I am thoroughly convinced that if they do it for one year, recording their progress, they will realize how much better off they are and not go back to their old ways. They will, in fact, become missionaries for the cause of good, healthy living.

We need to be focused on the *long-term benefits* of exercise. We are a people of instant wants and desires. Lose ten pounds in ten days. Drop three dress sizes in two weeks. Take a shot or a pill to build your muscles—all these things are a deterrent to good health and are certainly not answers.

The first thing we have to do is face reality, of course. For the average person who hasn't worked out or maintained a daily exercise regimen, your goals for the first thirty days should be that you exercise the days you say you will—*no excuses*—and that you do not hurt yourself. That's it. My rules are quite simple and quite easy. That's why I will accept no excuses. You are building good habits, and there's no reason for you to quit. At the same time, there are thousands of reasons (all inside your body) why you should continue.

Here is a list of suggestions to help the less motivated and further encourage those of you who have made up your minds to exercise.

**1.** Remember to write down your goals (the weight you'd like to reach; the time in which you'd like to walk, swim, or bike a certain distance) before you start anything else. First, begin with monthly goals for one full year, along with a plan for how you will put these goals into motion. Be sure to write down how you feel mentally, physically, and emotionally at the beginning and end of each month as you progress. You will begin to notice how much better you feel as you exercise more and more.

**2.** Decide which is the best exercise for you. My choice, and the logical choice for most beginners, is walking. It's inexpensive. It's good for your heart. It's good for your nervous system. It's good for your bones and muscles. It's even good for your mental health. Some people may choose joining a gym where they can swim or work out with weights. It's really up to the individual.

**3.** Have someone take a photograph of you before beginning your program. Allow the picture to show the real you. Take a photo in the same pose and wearing the same clothes each month so you can monitor your progress.

**4.** Keep written documentation of your progress. For instance, if you choose weightlifting, write down the type of lifting exercises you do, how much weight you lift, and how many repetitions you do. Note how much more you can lift and how many more repetitions you can do by the end of the month. If you choose walking, keep track of how far you walk and how long it takes to walk it. Good record keeping will help prevent you from lying to yourself.

5. Exercise by yourself. You've probably been told to do just the opposite, but if you have an "exercise buddy," he or she may quit and this may encourage you to do the same. You are doing this for yourself, so do it by yourself. Ultimately, when you are secure in your ability to stick with it, allow a friend to join you. It might even be more encouraging for you when you help someone else progress as much as you have.

6. Make the exercise fun. I promise you, it is possible. If you decide to walk, buy a portable stereo with a headset and listen to your favorite music while walking. If you lift weights, jump rope, or ride a stationary bike, join a gym where you can meet new people or work out in front of the television during your favorite programs. Do whatever it takes to make your workouts fun.

7. Nothing short of an oncoming tornado should come between you and your exercise time. Choose the time of day that you will exercise carefully before you start your program. Whatever time you choose, exercise at that time of day every day, even if you don't really feel like it. If you feel stressed, exercise will help alleviate some of that stress. If you are tired, exercise will rejuvenate you. If you do not feel well, exercise may help you feel better. If you are very busy, a break from work could do wonders for you. If necessary, shorten or minimize your workout. A little exercise is better than none at all.

As a chiropractor, I believe in practicing what I preach. I exercise regularly, I eat a nutritious, well-balanced diet, and I get regular chiropractic adjustments. I believe that overall health begins with a well-adjusted spinal column. In addition to correcting misalignments, I feel it is important for me to further advise and educate my patients on the positive benefits of regular exercise to help strengthen spinal muscles, which in turn, helps to reduce vertebral subluxations.

I am also firmly convinced that simply following an exercise program and getting periodic adjustments is not enough. Have you ever been to a gym and noticed that after vigorous exercise a person will light up a cigarette once they leave the building. This doesn't happen as much anymore because people are getting smarter, but it does happen. Most people who are "into health and exercise" have tossed the Marlboros out the window years ago, yet they will still stop at their favorite fast-food restaurant on their way home and pick up a burger and fries and a thick shake.

Just because you are following a good exercise program does not mean you can just run hog-wild through the fast food lanes. A Frosty is not a reward for swimming sixteen laps in the pool. Remember that, will you?

Most people hate to exercise—at first. Mark Twain once said that he got his exercise by walking to the funerals of his more athletic friends. Twain was an amusing man, of course, but we can hardly subscribe to his philosophy of exercise. Exercise is extremely effective. The trick—if there is one—is to begin small. Take a short walk. Do a few bends. Stretch. Try low-impact aerobics. The advice we most often hear is to try to exercise twenty minutes a day at least three days a week. We could all manage that, even if we were president of General Motors—or the United States—or a suburban mom (who is probably busier than both of them). Even the minimal amount of exercise offers rewards that are so important and so extensive that anyone who makes the effort to take that first walking step will soon become so acutely aware of its value that he or she will not consider it a chore but a privilege—and in time, a pleasure.

OK, so you don't think so now. Let's start slowly. Try it for just six weeks, exercising twenty minutes a day, three or four times a week. Make a note of your feelings. See if you don't feel much better. I'm hoping that in that length of time you will become addicted to exercise and do it, not because you think you should, but because you really want to.

You don't _have_ to exercise if you don't want to. But you _do_ have to, if you want to enjoy good health for any length of time. Not only will you feel better (check your notes), but if you stop, after awhile you will feel bad (check your notes again). We have some 650 muscles in our bodies, which interact with over 200 bones, and together they are responsible for our every movement. It takes forty muscles just to lift one of our legs. Our bones are living, breathing, porous structures with tiny blood vessels that have blood flowing through them. Our blood, in fact, is manufactured in the marrow of our bones at a phenomenal pace. It takes only a second for our bodies to lose about 3 million red blood cells, and it takes the same amount of time for us to replace them. One researcher (with little to do, probably) figured out that if the red blood cells in the body of one individual were stacked on top of each other, they would reach 31,000 miles into space. Granted, this is, for all intents and purposes, a useless piece of information, but isn't it absolutely amazing?

When the body goes into action, the response is that more blood is sent to the working muscles to help us complete whatever task we undertake. If we do not exercise, we become weakened, and the body's physical powers are greatly diminished. Your exercise routine should include cardiovascular or aerobic, strength, and flexibility training.

### Aerobic Exercise

The word "aerobic" means "with oxygen," which really doesn't tell you much, does it? Aerobic exercise involves much more than a Spandex leotard and those slim beautiful women hopping about on television. It is something that gets you perspiring and doubles your resting pulse rate for twenty to thirty minutes. This oxygenates the blood. Your capacity for this muscular work is dependent upon your supply of oxygen to your working muscles. Activities such as swimming, jogging, handball, basketball, bike riding, rope jumping, stair climbing, and many other athletic activities can be called aerobic exercises. Walking is also considered to be an aerobic exercise, but it usually demands a longer duration and brisk gait to be most effective.

## Can Exercise Hurt Me?

Exercise in some forms *can* hurt some people. It can, in fact, do a great deal of damage, and you should be aware of that before starting any exercise program. This is the reason why physically unhealthy people should learn their limitations from their chiropractors, and their medical doctors, if necessary.

Some chiropractors warn their patients about the effects of some forms of strenuous exercise on joints, ligaments, and the spinal column. Again, I must stress the words "moderation" and "common sense." Although jogging can reduce tension, improve the ability to deliver oxygen to all parts of the body, increase muscle tone, and improve blood circulation; it does jar the body, particularly the spine, and can actually cause vertebral subluxations. Other activities such as snow skiing, wrestling, and football often lead to strains in the spinal muscles and injuries to the spinal column itself. While chiropractors do not discourage patients from these forms of exercise and activities, we do suggest a complete spinal exam before beginning any physical sport to determine if there should be certain limitations. Also, if there is any mishap or injury of any kind during or after these activities, it is best to pay an immediate visit to your chiropractor's office.

## Chiropractic and Sports

Ask anyone who has been backstage at a concert or a television show or on a movie set or athletic field, and they will tell you that much of the real action and excitement is unseen by the audience. What you see on your TV screen or from the third row of an arena is only part of the story.

Television viewers of the Summer Olympic Games in Seoul, South Korea, in 1988, watched in horror as they saw gold medal winner Greg Louganis strike his head on the diving platform during the diving competition. What those behind the scenes saw was Jan Corwin, an American chiropractor on the Olympic Committee staff, give a spinal adjustment to Louganis immediately after the accident. Soon the fans saw Louganis return to the board and win another gold medal for the United States. They didn't know how he did it, only that he seemed to be all right after the incident.

When Dr. Tom Hyde, D.C., of Miami was appointed to the Olympic Committee medical staff for the 1987 Pan American Games in Indianapolis, it was a major boost for the chiropractic profession. It was not done, however, because the committee recommended it, but because the athletes themselves insisted that chiropractors be included among the staff because they knew firsthand how effective and helpful an adjustment could be for them.

Those in sports, both professional and amateur, are looking more and more to chiropractic care as an answer to their many problems. Chiropractor William R. Moyal, director of the Chiropractic Sports and Family Health Center in Pembroke Pines, Florida, was consultant to the 1988 United States Olympic Greco-Roman Wrestling Team. Dr. Moyal also takes care of forty of the members of the Miami Dolphins football team, has served as house doctor for the athletic department at Nova University in Fort Lauderdale, Florida and as a team chiropractor for local high school athletics. Dr. Nick Athens, D.C., has given chiropractic care to more than half the players on the San Francisco 49ers pro football team, including Joe Montana.

## NUTRITION: YOU *ARE* WHAT YOU EAT

You've heard the saying "you are what you eat." Maybe it should be amended to read "you *feel like* what you eat." Not only do chiropractors believe that good nutrition is a must, we believe that dietary intake of harmful substances such as toxins from alcohol, food additives, and pesticide residues in food are factors that can lead to subluxations of the spine, resulting in dis-ease in the body.

B. J. Palmer took an interest in nutrition long before it was "fashionable," but he warned that prescribing specific diets was "contrary to the basic philosophy of chiropractic." It was his belief that each person is unique, with unique dietary needs, and each person could intuitively choose the necessary foods if given the chance (once the subluxations were taken care of). His presumption was that our innate intelligence or common sense would tell us what our bodies needed and when they needed it. R. W. Stephenson, a professor at the Palmer College of Chiropractic, wrote, "the nourishment of the body should be governed by Innate Intelligence, with the cooperation of the educated mind," and that "the educated mind should serve as a cooperative function and not as a hindrance to the innate mind, in the selection of food for the body." Stephenson was also quoted as saying, "A sick person's abnormal educated mind will not allow him to use common sense; therefore, somebody else's common sense must be used."

Even in the early 1900s, several of the training colleges taught nutrition as part of their regular curriculum. Medical schools and other colleges operated under the assumption that nutrition was of minor importance. Fortunately, this attitude is changing somewhat—it is changing slowly, but changing, nonetheless. In a country where almost 15 percent of the population is considered to be 30 percent or more over their desirable weight, this attitude ought to be changing.

## America's Most Unwanted

If you read The American Chiropractic Association Council on Nutrition's "Ten Most Unwanted List," you might think you are looking at America's menu of the day. The ten most unhealthy things to partake of are as follows:

- White refined sugar and candy.
- Alcoholic beverages.
- Coffee.
- Cola beverages and artificially colored drinks.
- Artificially flavored products with preservatives added.
- "Junk food" and "snacks" (This covers a very wide range of products).
- White flour products.
- Hot dogs and most fast-food items.
- Tobacco.
- Pre-prepared foods such as TV dinners (high in sodium, fat, and artificial flavors or colorings).

So, what's for dinner tonight?

We all know our diets have become increasingly complicated considering all of the food additives now being used and America's growing food allergy problems. Many of today's farmers who run multimillion dollar farms and ranches cut corners everywhere they can, and one of the best ways is by using chemicals to kill the weeds, to make the crops bigger, to get more milk from cows, and so on. You won't see anyone out in the fields with a hoe getting rid of weeds anymore. Everything is done the "chemical way." There even used to be an advertising slogan that told us we were enjoying "better living through chemistry."

We cannot give up nor even become discouraged by the barrage of new information coming at us every day. Again, we just have to want to spend enough time to read and research to learn exactly what will enhance our health and what will harm it. We have to be smart enough to follow a selected food plan. We have to do this because it *matters*. It matters to our health, to our children's health, and to their children's health. If we say it doesn't matter, then there will be no generations to carry on after us—and then it really *won't* matter.

## Vitamins and Minerals

Do we *really* need to take vitamin and mineral supplements? No we don't. Not if we eat the perfect meal at every sitting, and if all the food we ingest is environmentally safe and poison-free. Do you do that? I didn't think so. So it is important to realize that you need those extra vitamin and mineral supplements for a healthy body and healthy bones. There is neither time nor space in this book for me to go into all the benefits of a good vitamin and mineral plan, but here are a couple of important points for you to consider.

When you consider that there are at least forty different nutrients—including protein, carbohydrates, fats, vitamins, and minerals—necessary to the human diet, we need to do more than just think about a proper diet, we should work hard to discover the right diet for our own individual needs.

If we look at the needs of the central nervous system alone, we can see how important proper diet and nutrition are to our bodies. While most of us are aware that too much fat in our

# Did You Know...

... that there is a widely held theory that animal products cause cancer? I refer to Harvey and Marilyn Diamond's *Fit for Life II—Living Health*. In this book, they certainly don't beat around the bush on this topic. "Animal products cause cancer. Absolutely no doubt about. It is not an issue of whether they do or not. They do!"

They believe the only issue is how large a part animal products play in our war with cancer. It is their contention that if all animal products were removed from our diets, cancer (other than smoking-related) would "cease to be a problem." They point out that it has already been proven "that because of their high-fat, high-cholesterol, low-fiber content, animal products cause their share of cancer, among which are cancer of the colon, breast, liver, kidneys, prostate, testicles, uterus, and ovaries."

When they tried to tell people about the link between colon cancer and diet years ago, no one was interested. More than fifty years ago, natural hygienists also warned of this link, but nobody listened to them either.

... that now, organizations such as the National Cancer Institute and the American Cancer Society are telling us that, yes, indeed, the link between what we eat and cancer is to be considered, and that colon cancer is one of the cancers that can be prevented by maintaining a good diet?

diets is extremely bad for our bodies, we may not realize that we need some fat. Fat provides essential fatty acids for the normal development of nerves, amino acids, and minerals that aid in normal nerve transmission. Try putting the wrong kind of fuel—or no fuel—in your automobile, and see how far you get. The wrong types of food can have the same effect on your body.

Certain B vitamins are important for healthy nerves, and thiamin is essential for proper nerve function; therefore, vitamin deficiencies can lead to illness in both the brain and peripheral nervous system. If proper nutrition is lacking, nerve conduction from the brain to the cells would be decreased and could be interrupted altogether. Also, if the intestines can't properly absorb the nutrients due to deficiencies, then this decreased absorption could disrupt sound body to brain to cell functions. Iron and certain amino acids are among the nutrients essential to this process. Children with iron deficiency often have a short attention span, as well as other behavioral and developmental problems related to a nervous system that is functioning poorly.

We have learned in recent years that certain elements have been found to have an adverse affect on the nervous systems of some individuals. Food additives containing vasoactive amines such as monosodium glutamate (MSG) have been linked to hyperactivity and severe allergic reactions in children as well as adults because of their effects on the central nervous system.

We also have to consider our all-important bones when we think of a complete diet. Calcium makes up some 99 percent of our skeletal structure, so it is a very important nutrient for maintaining the health of our bones. Osteoporosis, the loss of bone mass, can be due to a deficiency of calcium. Magnesium is important as a catalyst to help the body utilize the calcium. Phosphorus is also absolutely essential for bone strength.

Vitamin C is needed for the formation of collagen, present in connective tissue. Vitamin C is important in immune function and has been found to be essential for the healing of wounds and fractures. Because of vitamin D's role in bone mineralization, it is extremely important in maintaining bone density.

There are many excellent books on nutrition, written by people who have devoted years of research and effort into their projects, so there is virtually no excuse for us not to know what is good for us, regardless of the mass of confusion that abounds from time to time.

## COMMON SENSE

It is very difficult today to pick up a magazine or turn on the television without reading or hearing tons of new information about nutrition, exercise, and health. Unfortunately, what you read or hear about one day, may be changed the next week.

What was good for us before is no longer recommended, and what was considered a necessity for us as children is not only now passé but, in some cases, actually harmful.

Let's take a typical scenario for most of us. We open our evening paper to find a very persuasive, well-documented article that tells us that nitrates can cause cancer. Well, that's frightening. Later that week, perhaps in the same newspaper, we find another article, written by an educated person with many letters following his or her name, telling us that nitrates really don't cause cancer at all, offering strong evidence to support this case. Well, that's even *more* frightening.

Another magazine may offer an article that informs us that most of our water is polluted and harmful for us to drink—that it contains carcinogens, bacteria, and other dangerous pollutants. It cautions us to be wary of tap water and to purchase bottled water for drinking in order to be completely safe. Another article—this one written by an author with equally impressive credentials—warns us that bottled water in plastic containers may give off carcinogens, and water contained therein may not be nearly as healthy as we've been led to believe.

Well, good grief, what's a person to do? Many just say, "Hey, I'll do as I please, something is gonna kill me anyway. . . . I might as well go happy." Caffeine yes—Caffeine no. Sugar good—Sugar bad. Sugar substitutes are fine—Sugar substitutes cause cancer. Pork is good for you—Pork is bad for you. Drink your milk, honey, it'll give you strong bones—Don't give children milk, it's not good for them. Jog—Don't jog. Eat meat for protein—Avoid meat like the plague. A low-fat diet can save your life—A low-fat diet is extremely harmful.

Confused? Of course you are. And don't expect things to get any better. At the risk of sounding somewhat paranoid, I believe that there are some who want us to be confused, skeptical, doubting what we see and hear. I believe there are those in the medical establishment who want us dependent upon them. You may have reached the point where you do not know what to believe and feel it's impossible to sort out the rights and the wrongs.

There is one voice you can always listen to. It may not be as distinct as some of the other voices, and you may have to develop a relationship with this voice in order to decipher what it is really saying, but it is there. It's the voice of your own body. I have to revert back to the old common sense idea again. Your own body tells you how you should take care of yourself. We have to learn to be extremely selective about our choices, which, unfortunately, are growing every day.

I don't profess to be the smartest guy in the world, or even the smartest guy in Akron, Ohio, and I don't have all the answers. But I have done extensive research, talked to a lot of caring people, read many books, and tried and tested many theories; and I have found that common sense is still the best yardstick to use when measuring any kind of information.

When presented with a problem, I believe it is a good idea to examine it from as many angles as possible. See what kind of answers you come up with. It's all right, and often helpful, to seek the advice of experts, but who is more knowledgeable about your own body than the person who lives inside it? Not all of us have the same goals, attitudes, personalities, lifestyles, discipline, or body types. We cannot simply mix all the equations into a blender and come out with a glass of answers that "one size fits all." Listen to your own body talking to you. It talks to you all the time, whether you are listening or not. It never gives up on you, even when you have insulted, abused, or neglected it. Most of the time we just aren't trained to listen to what our bodies are saying, so we miss much of our bodies' wisdom as they try to help us. Relax. There's nobody in my head saying, "slay the king," or even "rob the liquor store," but I do believe we have our own built-in radar that is always honed in on our body's frequencies, broadcasting bulletins to our subconscious every second of the day. Let me offer a couple of examples.

Let's say you're 48 years old and thirty pounds overweight. You eat exactly what you want in any amount. You rarely, if ever, exercise. And, yes, you're ignoring all those naysayers who warn you about the harmful effects of cigarettes, and you smoke about a pack a day. Recently, you found out that you have high blood pressure, and even though you are concerned, you tell yourself that most people your age have high blood pressure, so what? Well, you are wrong. Most people your age do not have high blood pressure—that is unless they, too, are thirty pounds overweight, eat exactly what they want, don't exercise, and still smoke. A lot of those people are dead now from a stroke, lung cancer, heart disease, or some other illness related to their lifestyles.

What is your body telling you by elevating your blood pressure? That everything is all right? No. If you take the medication the doctor gives you, will the problem be solved? It will not be gone. Try stopping the medication, and see what happens. The blood pressure goes right back up. You have only treated the symptoms. It has been put on hold, but it is still on the line, waiting to take its toll on you. You have received fair warning.

Your body has tried, the best way it knows, to let you know that all is not well. You may also have shortness of breath, dizziness, and even an inability to do all the things you used to do. Well, I'm 48 years old, you say. No, that's not it. Your body doesn't care that you are 48. Your body cares that you are continuing to abuse and torture it, and it's trying its best to get you to listen. Does it have to give you a stroke to underscore its point a little better? I certainly hope not.

If you continue to allow the pressure in your blood vessels to rise long enough, one of these days the vessels will explode. If you don't heed this warning your body is giving you, you will be setting yourself up for major health problems in the future.

What can you do to help your body fight off this event? Number one, you can adopt a sensible diet. It's not hard to find one, they're in every book and magazine, and if you avoid the fads and "quick-fixes" you will find that most of them are well-planned. You will lose the weight that is burdening your body, and, as a result, lower the pressure in your blood vessels. Number two, you could stop smoking. Stopping won't kill you. I've heard people say they were "dying for a smoke" when they should have been saying, "I'm dying *from* a smoke." Number three, you can exercise. Stop groaning. I guarantee if you were to have a stroke, you would give all you own to be able to walk around the block again as you once could. And you *will* exercise then (if you survive), if not through your own volition, then through that of a physical therapist who will move your arms and legs for you. Am I being too harsh? Am I scaring you? I certainly hope so.

Another example would be if you were a 27-year-old female who had a baby six months ago. While carrying your child, your blood sugar level went much too high. You had some real bad days—but who doesn't when they are pregnant, right? And you experienced dizziness, nausea, fatigue, and headaches. Having a baby is no piece of cake, that's for sure. Besides, since the baby came you have been feeling much better. You're not feeling 100-percent well, but that will come, you keep telling yourself. At the same time, your body is warning you that something is still not quiet right. Oh well, you have work to do and a new baby to take care of. What are you supposed to do, go to your doctor and tell him or her that something is not quite right? He or she would just smile, pat you on the shoulder and tell you that all new mothers feel like this after the baby comes—it's just part of the package.

It's been proven that a woman who develops elevated blood sugar while pregnant has a very high risk of developing diabetes later in life. Her body is warning her that something is not working correctly. The stress of a pregnancy often brings out a weakness in the body that might not otherwise present itself. What is she supposed to do if she has these symptoms? The first thing she should do—and here I go again—is watch her diet. She should cut down on the number of soft drinks she consumes daily, lower her fat intake, and start a moderate exercise program. She may say she's too busy. She's a new mother, and she has the baby to think about. But would she like to see this child graduate from high school? Would she like to sit in the front row at her child's wedding? Would she like to cuddle her grandchildren? Of course, she would. Her body wants her to do this, too, and that is why it has sent out these little warning signals. Do something about your health. *Listen to your own body.*

I cannot stress enough the importance of taking responsibility for your own good health. Do your homework. Go to the library or bookstore, or talk to someone who understands good health and is an example of a healthy lifestyle. Do it right away. Tell yourself that this is the only body you have. It is the only one you will *ever* have here on earth, and you must take care of it, or it will not take care of you as you age.

If you are simply skipping merrily down the pathway of life thinking that everything will be all right, think again. In a world of excesses and environmental threats to our well-being daily, we must constantly be aware of our own bodies and of our responsibility to them.

I know that most young people think of themselves as invincible, but those of us who have taken a few steps ahead know better. Every day, we age a little more. We may not "get old," but we will get older. Someone once said that "the excesses of our youth are drafts upon our old age, payable with interest, about thirty years after date."

Amen to that!

# Chapter 12

# Is This War?

*In 1968, during the Vietnam War, a small company of American soldiers was marching through the rough, hot countryside, while nearing the end of a ten-day patrol. Suddenly, they were ambushed by the enemy. The point man took the full brunt of the attack. Everyone else ran, fell to the ground, and took cover. They were heavily outnumbered and outgunned. It looked hopeless.*

*The lieutenant in charge called to the downed point man, "Billy!"*

*At first there was no response. Then came a faint reply, "Help me. Help me."*

*Even though the jungle heat was intense, the men all felt a despairing chill as they exchanged looks of fear and anguish. It was then that the lieutenant became aware of another young man crawling up from behind.*

*"I'm going for Billy, sir," the young man said, without stopping.*

*"No, Johnny, don't," the lieutenant replied, as he put his hand out to hold the young soldier back. "You'll get killed if you try that. Don't do it."*

*Johnny managed a frightened smile and told his lieutenant that he had no choice. He began to crawl again in the direction of the voice.*

*"You can't save Billy, Johnny!" the lieutenant called out toward him. "It's not worth the risk. Come back."*

*Johnny could not hear him over the sound of heavy artillery and machine gun fire. It would not have mattered anyway. Nothing could have stopped Johnny as he crawled toward the place where Billy lay wounded and probably dying.*

*The rest of the company watched this tremendous act of courage, and they began to exert almost superhuman strength as they stepped up the firepower against the enemy. The battle seemed endless, but when it was over and the enemy had withdrawn, they were amazed that they were still alive.*

*They all rushed to the area where Billy was hit, hoping to find at least one, if not both, of them alive. What they found was Johnny lying across Billy's body. When the lieutenant gently lifted Johnny up, he could easily see that Billy was dead. He also discovered that while Johnny was still barely alive, he, too, was mortally wounded.*

*"Johnny, I told you not to try it," the lieutenant said, his voice trembling. "I told you it wasn't worth the risk. Billy's dead."*

*Johnny slowly opened his eyes, and with a serene look on his face, he managed to whisper, "Oh yes, sir, it was worth it."*

*"Don't you understand," the lieutenant said, leaning down so he could be heard. "Billy's dead."*

*"But he wasn't dead when I got here, sir," Johnny said softly. "He was alive . . . and he told me . . . he said . . . he knew I'd come for him. It was worth it all right."*

We all know that the truth is stranger (and harder to come by) than fiction. The truth is, without a doubt, something to be greatly desired, regardless of the circumstances. However, the truth is often at the mercy of those expressing it. One person's truth can also be considered another person's argument. The fact remains, however, that truth does not care who tells it—only that it's told.

Sir Francis Bacon once said, "There are three parts in truth; first the inquiry, which is the wooing of it; secondly, the knowledge of it, which is the presence of it; and thirdly, the belief, which is the enjoyment of it." In this chapter, I am going to present to you the truth as I know it. It is my hope that upon reading the facts presented to you in this chapter, you will not only come to believe the truth but will enjoy its benefits.

## I DECLARE WAR

I made the statement in Chapter 1 that there is a war going on between those in the medical profession and those who practice chiropractic care. "What are you talking about? Aren't you being just a little dramatic?" you may ask. No, I am not being dramatic at all. There is a David-and-Goliath-type war raging between the two sides. And though the influence of chiropractic is not as powerful as the medical profession's influence, I believe that, like David, we have truth on our side.

We are all aware that chiropractic is not a part of the mainstream in health care. That domain is owned—and fiercely guarded—by the medical profession. Over the years, other types of health-care professionals have managed to "sneak in under the wire," so to speak, and operate on the fringes, but the health-care system is a monarchy, with medical doctors occupying the throne. Chiropractors, as well as other alternative health-care providers, are a serious threat to the medical profession and to the large drug companies that support it. Their primary goal is to keep drug sales and profits up. It is a *business*, clear and simple. Now, we all know there is nothing wrong with running a business—it's how we all survive. But when dealing with another human being's health—or his or her life for that matter—we must prioritize in favor of the person who may be suffering or in danger of losing his or her life (as many medical doctors do).

It is frightening to even consider the possibility that certain segments of the medical profession do not want you cured of cancer, AIDS, heart disease, or other deadly illnesses. I know that you'd like to think that this idea is not only unbelievable but impossible. But, unfortunately, it *is* possible, and all too often, quite probable.

Prescription drugs are preferred by the medical community to less toxic, equally effective natural remedies. Narcotics and tranquilizers are advocated for the relief of pain instead of acupuncture, acupressure, massage therapy, stress reduction, chiropractic, or relaxation techniques. Furthermore, these alternative methods are not only suppressed when possible, but maligned and scorned by the medical community when they do manage to surface.

If you don't think that the medical profession is at war with chiropractic, ask your doctor about going to see a chiropractor. When one of my patients told his medical doctor that I had made the same diagnosis of his problem that the medical doc-

# *Did You Know...*

... that while it is true that some studies have found that taking aspirin can lessen your risk of heart attacks, it is also true that in these studies, the groups taking the aspirin had an increased number of strokes? The death rate was unchanged. So your real decision to make here is which one would you prefer to die from—a heart attack or a stroke?

tor made, the doctor didn't even bother to respond verbally. He simply walked out of the examining room and slammed the door, leaving the patient sitting cold on the table. This was intimidation at its very best—or worst.

## THE BATTLE PLANS

The battle plans of the American Medical Association (AMA) and the rest of the medical industry have been well laid, well thought out, and well-documented. The AMA's first tactic was to try to isolate the chiropractic-care field. In 1933, the Judicial Council of the AMA discouraged members from consulting with chiropractors or referring their patients to them for help. The stand taken by the AMA was quite explicit as stated in the following quote from a memo dispensed by the AMA: "The physician who maintains professional relations with cult practitioners would seem to exhibit a lack of faith in the correctness and efficacy of scientific medicine and to admit there is merit to cult practitioners." This "suggestion" was later changed to a "command." Any medical doctor who associated with a chiropractor was branded as unethical.

In 1963, the American Medical Association formed the Committee on Quackery for the sole purpose of destroying the chiropractic profession. An informant leaked documents and memos of the committee's meetings to the press and members of the chiropractic profession. It was revealed that this committee hired writers to pen anti-chiropractic articles and books to help destroy the credibility of the profession.

A confidential memo to the AMA Department of Investigation dated September 21, 1967, revealed the committee's short-range goals as quoted below:

1. Doing everything within our power to see that chiropractic coverage under Title 18 of the Medicare Law is not obtained.

2. Doing everything within our power to see that recognition of listing by the U.S. Office of Education of a chiropractic accrediting agency is not achieved.

3. To encourage the continued separation of the two national chiropractic organizations.

4. To encourage state medical societies to take the initiative in their state legislatures in regard to legislation that might affect the practice of chiropractic.

The long-range goal was to make chiropractic licensure so difficult that eventually more chiropractors would be dying than were being granted new licenses. Radiologists were also told that it was unethical to provide x-ray services to chiropractors and their patients. They were warned by the Radiological Society of New York that "a practicing radiologist in the State of New York shall have no voluntary association with cultists of chiropractic, including consultation and the acceptance of referrals."

Also according to the aforementioned memo, to further insure that "no new eggs would be hatched," medical organizations went into the high schools to insist that "no highly motivated and intelligent student be directed toward a career in chiropractic" because this would indeed be "a loss to society." A letter from the AMA to the president of the Pennsylvania Medical Society of Guidance Counselors condemned chiropractic as an "unscientific cult."

This is only a sample of the attempts made to discredit chiropractic. Why do you think the American Medical Association went through all the trouble of trying to get rid of chiropractic? Was it because they were so concerned about their patients falling into inept hands? No, that's not why. Was it because they didn't realize we were helping people? It wasn't that either. Did they think we were hurting people? They knew we were not hurting anybody. I believe they *knew* we were helping people. The real reason they wanted to get us out of their way was because they were afraid of us.

Any medical doctor with any sensibilities at all knows that the principle on which chiropractic is based is sound. They understand that the ground we stand on is a rock while theirs is sand, and it's crumbling. Many good doctors are frustrated by medicine's inability to heal the way it promises to. They are saddened by the fact that they cannot stamp out the growing disease and sickness that permeates our society. Chiropractic is attacked because the truth behind the theory of chiropractic will eventually topple organized medicine as we know it today. We have been fighting this war since the beginning, and we continue to engage in battle whenever and wherever we can.

The American Medical Association today boasts one of the richest and most powerful lobbies in Washington, spending more than $5 million in a typical election year to get those sympathetic to its causes elected to office. Yet, despite its phenomenal power and influence, its questionable tactics have not escaped the watchdogs. A number of legislators have openly and publicly expressed their disapproval.

Senator Edward M. Kennedy issued the following remarks in a 1971 address to his subcommittee on administrative practices:

> . . . Instead of the scientific and public professional organization it was founded as, the AMA has turned into a propaganda organ purveying "medical politics," for deceiving the Congress, the people, and the doctors of America themselves. The American Medical Association put the lives and well-being of American citizens below its own special interests in ordering its priorities. It deserves to be ignored, rejected, and forgotten.

## The Cold War

However, the war on chiropractic did not end back in the 1970s. It is still raging today, only it is much less subtle. It is more like a cold war. Today, the medical profession's tactics involve the dissemination of misinformation about chiropractic, not only to up-and-coming medical doctors, but to the American public as well.

A large percentage of medical doctors know absolutely nothing about chiropractic, and many refuse to be educated. Unless they have had the benefits of chiropractic proven to them firsthand, they have absolutely no clue about what we do. All they know is that we adjust the spine. That, however, is not *all* we do. They do not realize that we remove nerve interference through spinal adjustments. They do not realize how this helps the body to heal itself.

With the exception of those medical doctors who have become my patients, medical doctors rarely come to my office to see for themselves *exactly* what it is that I do. In my seventeen years of chiropractic practice, very few medical doctors, other than those who are my patients, have ever called and asked me questions about health-care choices or about any of my beliefs or knowledge about the health care of a patient. This is an example of the failure of an entire health-care profession to recognize the effectiveness and value of another health-care profession.

When those in the medical profession do come around and seek chiropractic treatment, I enjoy the reactions I usually get from them. I can almost predict what will happen. At first, they are extremely skeptical, wary, watchful, and sometimes even hostile. I am almost always their last resort, and they come because somebody in their family or circle of friends *insisted* they at least give chiropractic a try. So they come, sometimes just to prove to their family, friends, and colleagues that it will not work.

As the results overcome their skepticism, they become increasingly interested and ask many more questions than the average patient. It is great to see the changes made in their thinking as the changes take place in their bodies. They are often amazed at how chiropractic helps patients without drugs. Medical practitioners make great patients because they often take the time to inquire, study, and evaluate the treatment that is giving them relief when medicine had failed. Many of my patients are referred to me by those in the medical profession who have been under my care.

These medical practitioners learn firsthand that the misinformation they have learned about chiropractic is not true. If any of these negative charges were based on truth, then the first

100 patients who went to that first chiropractor 100 years ago would have spread the word about the uselessness of the procedures. Word of mouth is a powerful mechanism, and in those early days had a patient been harmed or not helped by the treatment, he or she would have bad-mouthed the chiropractor to all of his or her acquaintances. Soon there would have been no chiropractic profession at all. Chiropractic would have died a natural death and gone the way of so many of the so-called cures, fads, gimmicks, and treatments. Instead, the positive word has spread, and one of the things that has kept this profession alive and well today is the fact that chiropractic treatment *works,* and the people who are walking around with improved health are living proof that it does. Furthermore, they do not hesitate to tell everybody who will listen to them how much chiropractic has helped their condition. The simple fact is that chiropractic has millions of *satisfied* and pain-free patients. No wonder they keep nagging their friends to take advantage of treatment that they know firsthand is effective and drug-free.

One of the most asked questions in a chiropractor's office is "Why don't medical doctors believe in chiropractic care?" This usually comes from a patient who has gone to a medical doctor for years, yet has had years of pain. They had been subjected to numerous types of drugs, physical therapies, and surgeries, with very little hope of getting better. Suddenly, they find that they've been "miraculously" cured in the chiropractor's office. They then wonder why a chiropractor wasn't suggested by their medical doctor in the first place. Think of all the pain, deterioration, aggravation, and money it would have saved them.

While it is true that some medical doctors won't try to stop their patients from going to a chiropractor, they seldom suggest it, either. If their patients discover chiropractic care on their own, that's fine, but if they do not, that's fine too. That kind of logic is understandable to a degree. After all, does McDonald's tell you to run down to Wendy's if you want a good, thick milkshake? Does Wendy's admit that their coffee is not as good (or as hot) as McDonald's? Of course not. They did not become as successful as they are by referring their customers to another place.

If a patient does decide to see a chiropractor and tells his or her medical doctor, the response can be amazing. There are medical professionals who will actually tell you that "those people (chiropractors) will *hurt* you." I've had patients tell me that their medical doctors warned them to stay away from chiropractors because we keep asking our patients to come back, or they tell them that we claim to heal everything and prevent patients from getting the medicine they really need.

Do medical doctors ever tell you to come back to their offices? Do they prescribe (sometimes dangerous) drugs that you'll have to take for the rest of your life? Is this *OK?*

The most unfortunate thing about all of this is that many medical professionals really believe these fallacies to be fact, when they are nothing more than propaganda being spoon-fed to them by their medical educators, the American Medical Association, and other medical organizations.

Chiropractic has been referred to as an "unscientific cult," and chiropractors have been referred to as "charlatans," "quacks," and numerous other such names and charges, yet we have passed the test of time. Those who have been helped by chiropractic and are enjoying good health can readily attest to these facts.

Medical doctors can't always be blamed for their opinions and practices because they are merely reacting to what they've been taught to believe as fact. They, and the general public, are simply the unwitting victims of a sordid political campaign against chiropractic care that has been waged by the "lords of health-care organizations." Those involved in this campaign certainly feature the pharmaceutical companies. How could they possibly like chiropractic when we are a drugless health-care profession? We help and encourage people to get off drugs.

The American Medical Association has also succeeded in convincing the American public that chiropractors are a bunch of quacks and that medical doctors are the only *real* doctors. Dr. Richard E. DeRoeck gave a detailed account in his book *The Confusion About Chiropractors* of a going-away party thrown for him before his departure for chiropractic school. The highlight of the evening occurred, he said, when two of his friends presented him with a scrapbook that they had put together for him.

It contained a number of unusual cartoons and photographs taken from newspapers and magazines—two-headed creatures, witch doctors, Guinness Book oddballs—each accompanied by an appropriately comical chiropractic caption. Many hours of work had obviously gone into this most humiliating experience, and I had to remind myself that these were good friends, who were *on my side*.

While Dr. DeRoeck recognized that the parody was meant in fun, the scene, unfortunately, exemplified a common perception of chiropractic. He pointed this out by relating an experience he had with one of his early patients who was studying the certificates on his wall. "Why, I didn't know you went to *college*," the woman exclaimed in wonder. Did she think he just hung out a sign and pounded people on the back? Unfortunately, she probably did.

If you need health care, go to a medical doctor only. This has been the idea that the AMA has fed the general public for many years. And as far as many people are concerned, there is no other form of health care than medical care.

Chiropractors should not be too distressed that we have been selected as one of the American Medical Association's enemies. The AMA has openly opposed virtually every type of health-care profession that has come along and offered any kind of threat to its supremacy, including osteopathy, optometry, dentistry, and podiatry. The AMA has also gone on record as opposing many acts of social legislation that served the interest of public welfare such as Medicare, Medicaid, child labor laws, the instigation of the forty-hour work week, and minimum wage legislation.

I find it amazing that alternative methods of health care are held in such low esteem by the medical profession when, no longer than eighty years ago, medical education itself was regarded as disgraceful and shameful. Dr. Abraham Flexner, M.D., a well-known educator, was retained by the Carnegie Foundation to conduct a study of medical schools in 1910. His report "Medical Education in the United States & Canada" concluded that most of the 155 medical schools were merely "fly-by-night diploma mills that were only out after the tuition money." Of course, it is a well-publicized fact that the quality of medical education has been dramatically improved since this report. Unfortunately, the improvement that has taken place in chiropractic education and patient care has been a well-guarded secret.

Ann Landers, an advice columnist who has been referred to as the most influential woman in America, had been a frequent, and often vicious, critic of chiropractic care. Since her opinions and good common sense are widely respected, and her ethics seem to be without question, we can only suspect that she, too, had been misinformed and/or brainwashed to believe there is no real value in chiropractic.

I have to give the famous columnist credit, however, for her ability and willingness to present both sides of most arguments. She has recently stated in one of her columns that she has been accused of being strongly biased in favor of the medical profession, and she welcomed the opportunity to print a letter that gave a more balanced picture. She has since *recommended* chiropractic treatment after some inquiries from her readers.

She followed this column up with a series of columns that dealt with frightening statistics concerning hospital and medical safety. She also printed a letter from Theodore Babbitt, legal counsel for the Association for Responsible Medicine in Tampa, Florida, that offered more chilling statistics about the medical profession. He pointed out that in the *Journal of the American Medical Association,* a recent article stated that 64 *percent* of cardiac arrests at a teaching hospital were preventable. Another study of errors in a hospital intensive-care unit showed an average of 1.7 errors per patient. He went on to say that according to a Harvard Medical School study, negligent hospital treatment kills an estimated 180,000 Americans each year and injures *hundreds of thousands* more. Perhaps it might be a good idea to have a sign posted by the hospital doors reading: *"Caution, this building may be hazardous to your health."*

## Chiropractic's Battle Plans

Chiropractors treat only about 10 percent of the American population, which is twice as many as were treated by chiropractors in 1980, but that still leaves at least 90 percent of the population that does not have a clue about what we do and why. Even sadder is the fact that there are many who *think* they know what we do, but their information often comes directly from the medical profession and is often incorrect. Unfortunately, even the patients we treat are sometimes not very well-informed about their treatment. They only know it works, but they don't know how or why, and often they don't care.

Whose fault is this? The patient's? No. The medical doctor's? No. It's the fault of the *chiropractic* profession. As Walt Kelly's famous possum cartoon "Pogo" so aptly put it, "We has met the enemy . . . and he is *us.*" *He* (the enemy) is also the medical profession and the drug companies. It is understandable that those in the chiropractic profession might be wary of speaking up in light of what has happened in the past to those who have had the courage to extol the benefits of chiropractic treatment (as recently as the 1970s, chiropractors have been jailed for practicing their healing art), but we must continue speaking out about the health benefits of chiropractic.

I am extremely pleased that in the past few years chiropractors have been gathering courage to speak out and spread the word about the wonders of chiropractic. That is my primary reason for writing this book. I have always spoken out about the benefits of chiropractic to my patients and to those in my circle of friends, but I feel very strongly about the need to spread this word to a much larger audience.

We as chiropractors owe it to ourselves, and much more important, we owe it to our patients to spread the word about the potential for good health. We owe it to those who *should* be our patients but have been brainwashed to believe we can do them no good, and, in some cases, are actually frightened that we might harm them. The propaganda machine has done its work well, and it is up to us to set the record straight.

While it is quite true that the chiropractic profession has not done enough to educate the public on our own behalf, we are improving. We know that the general public opinion (that of those who have not experienced chiropractic care firsthand) simply reflects the negative propaganda being spread by the medical profession.

Although our public relations tactics are certainly lacking, I might add, in our defense, that many chiropractors still remember how intensely the AMA once harassed chiropractors in an effort to get rid of the profession. As mentioned previously, chiropractors were even jailed if they continued to practice. Due to this history, there is still some residual fear that we will be ridiculed even more or face even more dire consequences if we do tell the truth about chiropractic care and the wonderful things it can do for the body through the adjustment of the spine.

Since medicine has become a standard by which people often judge the education of health-care professionals, I will once again mention that that the rigors of training of medicine and chiropractic are quite similar. The only difference is that we study different types of subjects. Many people fail to realize that *chiropractic is not medicine*. Different education is required for different subjects; however, both are viable fields of study. It is not unheard of for one to have dual degrees and become a doctor of medicine and a doctor of chiropractic.

## SWEET VICTORIES

One of the more victorious battles of this ongoing conflict between medicine and chiropractic took place in 1976, when some chiropractors had taken all they could stand, and began to fight back. After a dozen years of enduring damaging propaganda, five chiropractors filed suit in a Chicago federal court charging the American Medical Association with unlawful restraint of trade practices and violation of the Sherman Anti-Trust Act. Three months later, a similar suit was brought to a New Jersey courtroom. Five months after that, more charges were presented in a Philadelphia federal court.

The war was indeed getting hot.

On August 28, 1987, U.S. District Court Judge Susan Getzendanner found the American Medical Association guilty of leading a conspiracy to destroy the chiropractic profession. The judge described the conspiracy as "systematic long-term wrongdoing with the long-term intent to destroy a licensed profession." The decision was appealed by the AMA, then taken to the U.S. Supreme Court in 1990. The Supreme Court refused to hear the case, thereby allowing Judge Getzendanner's decision to stand.

Five other defendants in that lawsuit, the Illinois Medical Society, the American Hospital Association, the American Osteopathic Association, the Chicago Medical Society, and the American Academy of Physical Medicine and Rehabilitation, settled in court earlier, affirming the right of chiropractors to engage in their profession.

Dr. Nathaniel Altman listed in his book *The Chiropractic Alternative* four major victories for the chiropractic profession that took place in 1974 as quoted below:

1. Louisiana became the last of the fifty states to grant a separate board of licensure [for chiropractic].

2. The Office of Education of the Department of Health, Education, and Welfare authorized the Council of Chiropractic Education (CCE) to begin accrediting training colleges.

3. Congress included chiropractic in its Medicare program.

4. Congress authorized a $2 million study on the scientific basis of chiropractic, which resulted in a landmark 1975 congress on The Research Status of Spinal Manipulative Therapy. This gave [chiropractic] practitioners equal status with other health care professionals.

Another interesting piece of information came out during the trials of chiropractic's lawsuits against the medical profession in the 1980s. Many medical doctors admitted that they had tried to practice chiropractic care on their patients. *The American Medical News* reported in January of 1981 that many physicians throughout the country were using "manipulative techniques similar to those used by chiropractors." Today, it is well known that many medical doctors are taking courses on manipulation of the spine because they know it works. You will also hear more and more medical personnel talk about natural health care. They want to be part of it because it is a better way of treating the patient. It is a better way of getting rid of disease and pain. It is a better way of health care. Isn't that what I've been saying all along?

There has been even more positive interaction between the medical and chiropractic professions in recent years, such as increased awareness of each other's professions and increased referrals between the professions, and this can only be good news for both professions, as well as for their patients. Though most medical doctors know little about chiropractic, whatever negative reports they have learned come from the medical educators and some medical publications. And the courts have proven that this information was not only biased but *specifically designed to destroy the profession,* not because it was an unfit profession, but because it was a threat to medicine's way of health care. So we really cannot blame the individual doctors for their misinformation. But this interaction between medical doctors and chiropractors helps members of each profession to learn more about the other, which helps to dispel medicine's incorrect notions about chiropractic and helps each profession to appreciate the other a little more.

Robert Mendelsohn, M.D., author of *Confessions of a Medical Heretic* and *How to Raise a Healthy Child in Spite of Your Doctor,* took a tongue-in-cheek perspective of the battle between the medical profession and chiropractors when he wrote the following: "I was taught in medical school never to 'consort' with chiropractors, but later was allowed to associate with them. Last year, as a result of the pressure of a lawsuit by the chiropractors, the American Medical Association allowed its doctors to consult with chiropractors. I predict at this rate, within a few years, M.D.s will be permitted to marry chiropractors."

## Dr. Henry Winsor, M.D.

It was more than fifty years ago that one medical pioneer, Dr. Henry Winsor, from Haverford, Pennsylvania, decided to investigate chiropractic care thoroughly. Dr. Winsor's studies took place in the early 1920s, when chiropractic was not only said to be ineffective but was considered, then more than ever, to be a "sham" or a "cult." For this reason, his study was extremely important, since he must have faced much opposition in his quest.

Faced with testimonies from patients who had experienced excellent results with spinal adjustments, he wondered how they could make such claims if there was nothing to them. He also wondered how the chiropractors could keep insisting that they could improve a patient's health if they could not back up their statements, but they often did.

"I wondered how chiropractors can claim such good results,"

Dr. Winsor wrote. "They claim that by 'adjusting' the fifth dorsal vertebra, between the shoulder blades, they can relieve stomach troubles and ulcers; by 'adjusting' a lumbar vertebra, they can relieve menstrual cramps; by 'adjusting' the fifth cervical, they can correct thyroid conditions and many other conditions; but how can they do that? We M.D.s criticize them, but *what if they have discovered a new, drugless way to treat disease?*" The italics are mine to emphasize this most important point.

*"What if they have discovered a new, drugless way to treat disease?"* Wouldn't it be great if all medical doctors asked themselves that simple question and kept an open mind about the answer? If we are to consider all aspects of care that relate to the good of the patient, this question has to be asked by medical doctors everywhere. If we pay any attention to any kind of studies at all, I don't see how anyone, medical or otherwise, can ignore the findings that Dr. Winsor presented.

It was after his graduation from medical school that Dr. Winsor was inspired by chiropractic and osteopathic literature to perform an experiment. He wanted to dissect human and animal cadavers to see if there was any relationship between the diseased internal organs discovered during the autopsy and the vertebrae from which the nerves that went to those organs originated. Dr. Winsor pointed out that the object of the dissections was to determine whether or not any connection existed between minor curvatures of the spine and diseased organs.

Dr. Winsor reasoned that if the chiropractors were right in their theory, then a misaligned vertebra that impinged a nerve going to the kidneys, for example, could weaken the kidneys and cause kidney disease. He also knew that if the theory was incorrect, then a misalignment in the "kidney place" of the spine would not find any corresponding problem in the kidneys themselves.

The University of Pennsylvania granted Dr. Winsor permission to carry out experiments on the subject. In a series of three studies, he dissected a total of seventy-five human and twenty-two cat cadavers. The results of his studies are as follows:

221 structures other than the spine were found diseased. Of these, 212 were observed to belong to the same sympathetic (nerve) segments as the vertebrae in curvature. Nine diseased

organs belonged to different sympathetic segments from the vertebrae out of line. These figures cannot be expected to co-incide . . . for an organ may receive sympathetic filaments from several spinal segments and several organs may be sup-plied with sympathetic (nerve) filaments from the same spinal segments.

The results showed an overwhelming (nearly 100 percent) correlation between "minor curvatures" of the spine and dis-eases of the internal organs including the stomach, lungs, liver, gallbladder, pancreas, spleen, kidneys, prostate, bladder, uterus, and heart.

The results of this impressive study were published in the respected medical journal *The Medical Times* and can be found in any medical, and some public, libraries.

Dr. Winsor was certainly not alone in his findings since sim-ilar studies by numerous other researchers over the next few decades would confirm his initial conclusion that a well-aligned spinal column is essential for a healthy body.

Do you realize just how important Dr. Winsor's findings are? This is a medical doctor talking. He is giving you *positive proof* that chiropractic care is an effective treatment—equal to, and often surpassing, the efficacy of medical treatment. All of this is accomplished without drugs or surgery. This study verifies and validates what chiropractors have been saying from the be-ginning. Chiropractic adjustments do more than relieve back pain. Chiropractic spinal adjustments can help the entire body be free from sickness, disease, and pain.

It is interesting to note that there have no been more stud-ies of this kind done since Dr. Winsor's study. Given such im-pressive results, one would think that those in the medical pro-fession would sit up and take notice or conduct another study in an effort to disprove Winsor's findings. Unfortunately, they have done neither. The medical profession does not want to ac-knowledge the impact of Winsor's study.

## Acceptance

There is some good news that comes from a report printed in the April 3, 1981 issue of *Medical Economics* noting that the percentage of medical doctors who refer patients to chiropractors has doubled since 1975. This is proof to me that medical doctors are caring more about the overall health of their patients and less about themselves and being the top dog.

Today, when people ask me why chiropractors aren't recognized as part of the mainstream health-care providers, I answer their question with a question: "Chiropractors aren't recognized *by whom*?" The answer is the American Medical Association. If you ask who *does* recognize the chiropractic profession, I can give you that answer as well: workers' compensation boards, Medicare, Medicaid, state governments, the federal government, insurance companies, and more and more patients every day.

I will also note here that some insurance and workers' compensation companies that had originally shunned chiropractic have done a complete about-face in their recognition of chiropractic's value when it was discovered that enormous amounts of dollars were saved by those claimants who sought chiropractic care. These patients' recovery- or "going-back-to-work-time" was cut in half. Do you realize that for the financial cost of just one back surgery, a patient could go to his or her chiropractor for treatment three times a week for more than four years?

Anyone thinking with a logical mind would wonder why there is any opposition to chiropractic, since it is certainly a reasonable, sensible, and drug-free approach to health care. In fact, the only harm it seems to do is to organized medicine's pocketbook.

## MY TREATY

It is my belief that both professions could greatly benefit from each other's knowledge and practices. Even more important, the people whose lives are on the line desperately need us to find some type of common ground. Chiropractors and medical doctors should try harder to work together for the benefit of the patients' good health. This is why I have outlined the following treaty to stop this war and correct the misinformation about chiropractic that is still being distributed to the general public.

- Medical doctors and doctors of chiropractic should work to-

# Did You Know...

... that health care in the United States cost $462 billion in 1986? In 1989 the total estimated health-care cost soared to $600 billion, or $19,000 a second. If the rate of health care costs continues to rise in this fashion, it will equal our current gross national product by the year 2040. Must we do something different? Of course we must!

gether for the betterment of the health of everyone. If medicine had all the answers, we would all be much healthier already, wouldn't we?

- Chiropractors should continue to be a totally separate and distinct professional entity from medicine. After all, why would we want to duplicate failure? A recent encounter I had with a patient is typical of many conversations that I have had with patients.

"Dr. Gandee, you didn't do anything like my medical doctor did."

"Are you here because what your family medical doctor and what the specialists did made you feel better?" I ask. "Or are you in pain?"

"No, I still hurt . . . nothing helps."

"Then why would you want me to do the same things to you that your medical doctor did, when they didn't help you?"

"I don't know."

This patient, and others before him, begin, at this point, to reach that first plateau of understanding. The first thing they have to learn is that chiropractic is an entirely different approach to good health. Very few things are more satisfying to me than seeing the light go on in a patient's mind breaking through years of misconceptions that have been offered to the general public about chiropractic care.

- Chiropractors should be permitted access to all hospital facilities. We need hospitals. Only a fool would fail to recognize the importance of a facility where people can receive specialized treatment. But the patient deserves *every available treatment* to help him or her survive. One of those treatments is chiropractic. I believe that it is very important for the patient to have access to chiropractic care, which turns the life force back on, and allows him or her to heal sooner and avoid as much suffering (and painkilling drugs) as possible. Chiropractic can do this, and until this becomes an accepted fact and chiropractic is available to all patients in all hospitals, the patient will be shortchanged.

• People should be encouraged to seek chiropractic care *prior* to medical care, rather than as a last-chance effort, when all else has failed. Sometimes, too much damage has already been done to the body, and chiropractic or any other form of health care, cannot undo it.

Chiropractic first. Drugs second. Surgery last. Doesn't this make sense to you? If you are a chiropractic patient, it certainly does. Chiropractic doesn't hurt people as the "old medical tales" would have you believe. There are no side effects to chiropractic treatment. There are side effects and danger with all medications. There are certainly side effects—and some fatal effects—with surgery. You can never undo what surgery does to your body. You can't put back what the surgeon takes out. When nerves, muscle, and tissue are cut, they will never be the same. Your body reacts to any kind of surgery with total shock because it is not what nature intended. The body knows what's good for it and what isn't. I know that there are times when surgery is a necessity, but that is the exception rather than the rule. People ought to try chiropractic first!

A big problem I see daily in my office is the patients who try chiropractic as a last resort. They've been to medical doctor after medical doctor for years and years. They've swallowed a truckload of drugs. They've gritted their teeth and tried to live with their illness as best they could, often settling for half of a life instead of the good health they deserve. They come to me because somebody told them I *might* be able to help. It pains me to see how much suffering they've already endured and how much damage—some of which can no longer be reversed—has been done to them in the name of "getting well." And are they well? Not by a long shot.

Before patients try chiropractic, usually they have first been everywhere, tried everything, and done all they've been told to do. They finally reach a point where they are totally frustrated, fed up, and plain old medicine-weary. And bless their sometimes-failing hearts, they are still sick. Some are even sicker than when they started. By the time we get them, their bodies are almost always showing a great deal of deterioration and degeneration. This is why I stress, again and again, chiropractic should be tried *first*.

- Insurance companies should require people to get a second opinion from a chiropractor, prior to just about every type of surgery. This is another example of the use of common sense. With statistics screaming at us that 80 percent of all surgeries are unnecessary, why on earth would any patient fail to explore other alternatives before submitting to the knife? It is utter foolishness to allow this kind of thing to go unchallenged. If chiropractic care can't help a patient, he or she can still elect to have surgery because chiropractic care does not harm the body, nor does it cause subsequent surgery to be ineffective. The same cannot be said about surgery, however. Once that scalpel cuts into your body, you cannot undo its effects.

Let's get our priorities in order. I'm talking about our lives, our health, and our overall well-being. This is not a decision to be taken lightly. These days anyone who does not check out all the health-care alternatives opens him- or herself up to a lot of pain and agony.

- Grade school, junior high, and high school health classes should teach *real* health not just how to brush your teeth and to change your underwear.

- Too many of those involved in the medical profession are too concerned about the money and not concerned enough about good health. Too many people in control of our health-care system are not even medical people. They are money people. They do not have the best interests of the people at heart. They look at health only as a business. The legal drug business is one of the most profitable industries in the world.

- Chiropractors should be as involved in health-care decision- and policy-making as medical doctors are. This will help insurance companies and federal agencies see alternative possibilities in health care.

- Legal drug commercials are contributing heavily to the illegal drug addiction problem that keeps growing in our country, in spite of all we try to do. The theme on television commercials is always the same. If you feel bad, then take drugs, and you will feel good! We have become conditioned to the "quick fix."

Is this the message we want to send to our children? Drug abuse of all kinds is all too often seen as necessary, sometimes fashionable, and sometimes "really cool." When a child is subjected to the notion that "drugs make things better" at a very early age—You're not feeling well? take this pill, and you will feel better—then we are sending a very strong message to them. Not only are they at risk for the legal drugs that can destroy a system, but they may not always learn the difference between "bad drugs" and "good drugs" (or drugs that are not quite as bad.)

What it all boils down to is that we are teaching our children that drugs make you feel good, and that's exactly what the drug companies want you to believe. It is horrific to even hear the suggestion that pharmaceutical companies don't want you well, but you should realize by now that this is true. They want you to have symptoms so you will use their products. They do not like chiropractic because we help you get well without drug therapy.

Think of the billions and billions of dollars drug companies spend each year trying to get you to see the effectiveness of their product and what it can do for you and your children. We've got to turn this message around. We must make it clear that drugs are *not* something fantastic that we take at the drop of a hat but for use only in extreme circumstances and *in moderation.*

- Although I believe in striving for a drug-free health-care program, I realize that some drugs are necessary, and even life-saving, in some cases. However, I believe medical doctors should *not* prescribe medication. (Oh, now I've done it!) The doctor should *diagnose* the problem and a pharmacist should, in conjunction with the medical doctor, prescribe the medication that the patient should take. And these drugs should be *severely* limited, monitored, and controlled. The primary reason for this belief is that medical doctors do not have the time to read up on every drug on the market today. They find themselves in the position of having to rely on the drug companies' salespeople who come to their offices offering free samples and incentive programs to increase the use of their drugs. In my opinion, medical doctors are not fully capable of both diagnosing a condition and prescribing the best drug for that condition because of the massive influx of new drugs coming into the marketplace every day.

  Do we really want to put our lives and our good health in the hands of a drug salesperson? We might buy a used car from a salesperson, or we may even try out a vacuum cleaner from one. But is it a good idea to gulp down a handful of pills that have been given to the doctor by a person with no medical training and who works on commission?

- Americans should receive *free care* when sick. Yes, I believe when you are sick, you should be able to go to your doctor and be treated for free! I believe the only time you should have to pay your doctor is when you are healthy! As long as you feel good, you should pay your doctor a regular monthly payment. After all, isn't that what we want our doctors to do—to keep us healthy? It would be worth the money, wouldn't it? Instead, we are getting what we pay for—sickness. If we received free health care when we were sick and paid only when we were well, there would be a whole new concept in preventative measures. Think about it. Isn't this like insurance? We pay for it when we're well, then when we get sick, it pays us. As long as we pay for sickness, I guarantee you, we will continue to get our money's worth.

- Change is stimulating. We can change our health habits very quickly, once we search for and understand *the whole truth.* To simply exist is not enough when there is truly a better way. I want to know what I can do *now* to enjoy a healthier old age. I want to know what I can do *now* to avoid all those horrors currently associated with getting old. I want to know what I can do *now* to assure myself and my loved ones that I will be a happy old man with a clear mind and the energy and enthusiasm to live out my last days with enjoyment.

## WHEN WILL THE WAR BE OVER?

When will the war be over? I really do not know. There is a cease-fire in some quarters, and the battleground is not nearly so strewn with casualties (the chiropractors and the suffering patients), but, as Casey Stengel says, it is not over until it's over.

It will finally be over when those in the medical profession are better educated in the ways of chiropractic and other alternative health-care methods and are able to fully give credit, recognition, and respect to an important segment of health-care professionals. Chiropractors have long known and accepted the important role of the medical profession, and we ask only that this be returned in kind.

The real winners in this unnecessary and ugly war will be those people who are seeking the best quality of health care from a complete spectrum of professionals whose only concern will be the total well-being of the patient.

If chiropractors can keep patients from falling into the swirling waters of disease and sickness in the first place, then there will not be so many that will have to be rescued. And what would well patients do with all that spare time and money once they are no longer spending it all at the doctor's office?

They can enjoy their good health! What an *amazing* concept!

# Chapter 13

# Adjusting Your Attitude

The old rancher stood beside his fence on his homestead just along the outskirts of the little community where he lived. On this day, as in the past, he watched the approaching covered wagons heading west in search of a better life. Sometimes the drivers would stop and talk for a while. Some would tarry long enough to eat a meal, while others would simply drive by and wave. As he stood there on this particular day, one of the wagons pulled up in front of him and stopped.

"Say, old timer," the driver called out to him, "Me 'n' my family here have come all the way across the country looking for a nice place to settle down. Can you tell me what kind of place this is and what the people are like who live here?"

The old rancher studied the wagon driver for a moment, then asked what the people were like in the place where he'd come from.

"Mean-spirited and hateful," came the caustic reply. The man's wife leaned out of the wagon and emphasized his assessment by saying that was one of the reasons they left. "Sorry bunch of people, they was," the man added. "Never a good word from nobody." They went on to say how happy they were to be gone from that terrible place. And the wagon driver's wife repeated the question. "What kind of people you got around here?"

The old rancher shook his head slowly before answering. "They're just like that here," he finally replied. "They're mean-spirited and hateful. I don't think you'd be happy here at all."

"Much obliged to you, stranger," the driver said, slapping the reins on his horses and clacking his tongue for them to giddy up. The wagon disappeared in a cloud of dust.

*Before long another wagon came into sight and, upon reaching the old rancher, stopped.*

*"Howdy stranger," the driver called out to him.*

*The old rancher tipped his hat and responded in kind.*

*"We've come out west to seek a better life, and we are looking for a place to settle," the wagon driver said. "What kind of people live around here?"*

*The old rancher studied the family in the wagon for a moment, as he did the occupants of the previous wagon. "What kind of people did you leave?" he asked.*

*"Fine, wonderful people," came the enthusiastic reply.*

*The man's wife leaned out from the opening in the wagon, and there was great sadness on her face. "Times was bad, mister, and the crops failed year after year," she said in a soft voice. "But we didn't want to leave 'cause we loved the people there so much." She went on to tell the old rancher that she and her husband and the kids were extremely sad for having left the people they loved, but they needed to search for a better way of life.*

*"Yep, the folks we left were all wonderful people," her husband said. "But we hoped we might find fine folks out here as well. What kind of folks did you say lived around here, mister?"*

*The old rancher smiled. "Why, they're fine, upstanding people, " he answered. "Wonderful people. You'll like them—and they'll like you. Fact is, I'll wager they're just like the ones you lived around before. I think you've found just the place you've been lookin' for."*

Too many people are unaware that about 90 percent of their quality of life is governed by their attitudes. One with the mindset that all will be terrible and that everything will go wrong is usually not disappointed. The same goes for that person who is forever seeing rainbows, bluebirds, and roses. They will always be able to enjoy that which has been put here for us to embrace.

In my office I make adjustments to the back, but I make no claims to making any kind of attitude adjustments. That part is up to you. Now, you may think your attitude depends upon your surroundings. *If* you have a good job, *if* you have a good spouse, *if* you have good children, *if* you had good parents growing up, *if* you are in good health—then you can have a good attitude. If, if, if. None of this is true, of course. Those who have the most going for them often are the most miserable of human beings, and those who appear to have little often seem to be able to smell the flowers and enjoy life.

So I have to come to the conclusion that it's not what you have or even who you are that governs your attitude, it's how you feel about life that makes a difference. I think we'll also agree that a healthy person is often a happy person. Considering the fact that I believe chiropractic offers you a much better shot at good health than any other health-care system, I would have to say that perhaps I am *somewhat* responsible for attitude adjustments in my office.

Those in the real estate business are fond of saying that only three things count when looking for a home to purchase: *Location, location,* and *location.* This might be amended to say that only three things count in what you make of your life: *Attitude, attitude,* and *attitude.*

The same is true of health. Attitude definitely plays a very positive role in overall health—both in prevention of illness and recovery from illness. Did you know that pessimists suffer *twice* the number of infectious illnesses as optimists? The amount of time it takes an optimistic patient to recover from an illness is usually much less than the amount of time it takes a pessimist to recover. According to an article in the August 1997 issue of the journal *Arteriosclerosis, Thrombosis, and Vascular Biology,* middle-aged men who expressed high levels of despair had a 20-percent greater rate of atherosclerosis than their more optimistic counterparts.

How many books can you name that offer various themes on this concept? If we were playing a trivia game, the answers could go on and on. One of the best-selling books of all time comes to mind—*The Power of Positive Thinking* by Norman Vincent Peale. Journalist Bill Moyers in the 1994 PBS television documentary entitled *Healing and the Mind* placed great emphasis and importance on attitude or state of mind in the healing process of chronically ill patients. Norman Cousins also attributed his healing process primarily to a positive attitude mixed generously with humor and laughter in his book *Anatomy of an Illness.* Another of the best-selling books of our time *How to Win*

*Friends and Influence People,* written by Dale Carnegie, bases its entire premise on a positive attitude. Readers of the book, plus the thousands who have taken the course of the same name, tell life-changing stories about how the positive approach has made the difference between despair and happiness in their lives. It has created success in their professional and personal lives and general good health.

## APATHY

Apathy is extremely dangerous to your attitude. It is probably the best description of a bad attitude. According to *The American Heritage Dictionary,* it means "lack of emotion or feeling." It is an indifferent or insensible attitude. When one is adamant in his or her beliefs or opinions, at least you have a chance of discussing or even arguing your point with him or her. Apathy offers no room for discussion because the person simply does not care. Most people have lapses of emotion sometimes or a certain amount of frustration to the point where we *say* it doesn't matter to us what happens, but we seldom mean it, and we usually snap out of it somewhat quickly. However, when this type of thinking becomes a philosophy of life, it becomes a problem.

Not too long ago, I saw a bumper sticker that read "Tomorrow has been canceled, due to lack of interest." The statement is made with a wry sense of humor, but isn't it a little frightening as well, especially since it is so applicable to our society today? Another gem is the joke that has one fellow asking another if he thinks that most of the problems in the world today stem from ignorance and apathy. The second man replies, "I don't *know* . . . and I don't *care.*"

## WHEN IT'S YOUR TIME . . .

Many also hold the defeatist attitude that everything that *can* go wrong *will* go wrong—at the *worst* possible time. It's supposed to be "Murphy's Law," but it's an extremely negative way to look at life. It would be better to say that everything that *can* go right *will* go right—at the *best* possible time. Have you ever heard anybody say that?

I'll bet you've never heard anyone who just won a large amount of money or had something wonderful and unexpected happen to them exclaim, "Oh, that's *just my luck!*" No, they use that phrase when something terrible happens, meaning, of course, "my *bad* luck." When the people from Publisher's Clearing House pull up to a house in their cute little van, almost all of the prize winners yell out, "I can't believe it!" I long to see just one contestant open the door and say, "Hey, where have you guys been? I've been waiting for you. I *knew* you would come." Well, all right, that may never happen, but it's amazing how we always accept good news with astonishment and bad news with the resigned attitude of "I *knew* it would happen."

I'm sure you've also heard people say, "When it's your time, you'll go; otherwise it's not your time." A friend of mine who worked as a civilian writer for the U.S. Air Force recruiting department remembered an incident wherein two sergeants did not want to fly to and from their destinations with their captain, who was to be piloting the plane. His skills in the cockpit were not skills you'd want to bet your life on, they insisted. When someone mentioned to one of the sergeants that they should not be worried about flying with the captain, in spite of his poor piloting skills, because "when it is your time to go, you'll go; and if it isn't, you won't, so don't worry," One of the sergeants replied, "Yeah, but I don't want to be with *him* in that plane, when it's *his* time to go."

Even though it is a possibility that we have allotted times upon the earth, it would appear that we can ask for life extensions from our Creator, otherwise prayer and meditation would be unnecessary. There are promises in God's word that offer us a chance for longer—or shorter—lives. Many people shorten their allotted time by mistreating their bodies, neglecting and abusing their health until their bodies can no longer put up the good fight. We have choices in life, and how we choose to live our lives is our responsibility. We are free, indeed, to make our own choices, even poor ones. If you believe in a creator, you must also believe that this creator is able to extend your time on earth, and you must use the common sense you were given at birth to get your time extended.

# *Did You Know...*

... that smoking is more costly to your health than heroin, cocaine, or alcohol? More people die from smoking-related illnesses each year than from AIDS, car accidents, alcohol abuse, homicides, fires, and suicides combined.

... that cigarette smoke contains more than 3,000 chemical substances?

... that a pack of cigarettes a day increases the risk of a heart attack two-and-a-half times? Yet the amount of money spent annually on smoking advertisements has increased from $3.13 billion in 1985 to $5.23 billion in 1992. Only automobile manufacturers advertise more than tobacco companies.

... that smoking-related illnesses kill more than 400,000 Americans each year? That's more than 33,000 a month. Can you even imagine more than 1,000 dead people daily because of an addiction to a gross and disgusting habit that fouls your breath, burns holes in your furniture and clothes, and stains your teeth. Ask yourself this question: Is it really worth a puff?

## QUALITY OF LIFE

Life without good health is a life of poor quality, regardless of your standing among your family members, in the community, or in the world. Poor health does not care if you have millions of dollars in the bank, own a chateau in the South of France, have naturally curly hair, or drive a pale blue Rolls Royce. Actually, poor health does not care about you at all, and you must approach it the way you would approach any other enemy. Fight against it with every weapon available to you.

It is also important not to wait until poor health has you in its deadly grip with a strangulation hold on your already weakened body. Fight it before it breaks through your fortress walls and disposes of your defensive troops. In Chapter 5 I discussed how our immune systems stand guard to keep us out of harm's way. But those scrappy little defenders sometimes need help—

and lots of it. What kind of help? Positive reinforcements from a positive attitude.

I certainly hope that by now you are convinced that you are a wonderfully designed machine, capable of far greater achievements than you might ever have believed possible. You cannot deny that our bodies are walking, talking, thinking, breathing miracles. Think about it. Human-made machines such as the phonograph, the computer, the automobile, and the airplane are all impressive, to say the least, but think of your own functioning body and how beautifully it was designed to serve us here on earth.

Unfortunately, we are living in a war zone. No, I am not talking about the daily news reports of drive-by shootings, spousal and child abuses, robberies, rapes, and murders. I am talking about the constant threat of debilitating illness and disease. Nothing brings home the reality of unbearable suffering more than the growing support for the doctor who advocates assisted suicides. When the general public prefers the services of Dr. Death over the services of someone who is trying to help him or her or a loved one fight a horrible illness, something is terribly wrong. Will there be a time when we refer to a health "don't-care" system? Are we already there?

There have been studies done with both children and adults with terminal diseases showing what can be accomplished through visualization procedures. This concept—telling someone to imagine a bunch of little bad guys inside his or her body seeking to destroy him or her, and he or she must then conjure up this group of "good guys" to take them down in defeat. However, many patients who have tried using this type of imagery have gone into what medical doctors call spontaneous remission. Medical doctors say they do not understand it, but something happened.

What happened? I cannot say for sure. I cannot prove that their positive thinking caused the remissions of their diseases anymore than the naysayers can prove that it didn't have a hand in it. The doubters are almost always those who have not been faced with such a crisis and fail to realize the amazing power of our own brains (with a little help, of course, from a higher power).

In a 1988 study conducted by C. D. Cayce, students were divided into three groups. One group worked on crossword puzzles, the second group was given relaxation training, and the third group received relaxation training plus visual imagery training, in which they pictured their powerful and strong immune systems attacking weak cold and flu viruses. Was there a difference in the groups? Group one showed no increase in immune cells. Group two showed a slight increase. Group three showed a significant increase after only one hour of training.

It's obvious there is a lot to learn about health, but we are not going to learn it from the current leaders of our health-care system. In basketball, coaches constantly remind the players to see the ball going into the basket before they shoot. At home and on the court, they tell them to just close their eyes and play a game in their minds and watch the ball go exactly where they want it to go. This can work in all aspects of life. If you just visualize yourself going where you want to go in life, you can get there. Sometimes all it takes is a little positive thinking. Sometimes all the positive thinking and upbeat attitude in the world may fail to work, but our attitude does play a great part in what happens in our lives.

I am reminded of an incident that happened a few years ago at a bicycle race in Medina, Ohio. At the end of the race, some of the participants were discussing all the reasons and excuses for why they hadn't done well. The excuses were varied. One's bike didn't hold up, another said someone was blocking him on purpose, another had a cramp in his leg, and there were several other reasonable excuses. One rider shook his head and talked about how he had been doing extremely well. He was way ahead of all his friends and was, in fact, feeling quite proud of himself, when he was almost "blown off his bike" by another cyclist who passed him in a flash. It so unnerved him that he ended up dropping out of the race altogether.

"Hey, that happens," one of the other riders said, slapping him on the back. "There's always somebody out there who is faster than you. He probably had some kind of an edge—you know how that is."

"Yeah, this guy had an edge, all right," the man admitted reluctantly. "He only had *one* leg."

The guy with one leg was Kyle Underwood from Norton,

Ohio. The young man had lost his right leg to bone cancer at the age of twelve. He later went on to the ParaOlympics in Seoul, Korea in 1988, where he would come in fourth in the international games. It would have been easy and understandable for him not to have participated in the race at Medina, or even to not ride a bicycle at all, but Kyle had always felt that his best training would be to enter races where able-bodied cyclists competed. That way, he would be forced to push himself just a little harder. On this particular day, in a field of more than 200 participants, none of whom were physically challenged, Kyle finished in the top twenty. Was it the extra strength in his remaining leg? That helped, of course, but I tend to think it had a lot to do with attitude—the sincere belief that *he could do it.*

What excuses do you have for not doing what you want or need to do?

## STRESS

It has been said that stress is simply a reaction to something life offers us. Some people face major negative changes in their lives, jobs, families, finances, or health head on, tackling them with a positive attitude, while others are totally destroyed by any negative happening. It's not *what* happens to you, but how you react to what happens to you that makes all the difference. Once again, it all depends on your attitude.

We are often overwhelmed in today's world by the constant stress that surrounds us. Actually, another word for stress is often "life." Grandma Moses, the American painter who lived to be 100 years old and who obviously handled stress quite well, has been quoted as saying: "Life is what we make it—always has been—always will be." Hardly profound, but true just the same.

It is usually not stress—especially the everyday kind—that does us in but our *reaction* to the matter at hand. Some stress is not bad at all. Some of it is even a motivator, something many of us need in order to get things done. Schedules, appointments, deadlines—they all serve to get things moving.

Another excellent observation of humanity comes from Bernie Siegel, M.D., in *Love, Medicine, and Miracles*: "It is often said that stress is one of the most destructive elements in people's daily lives, but that's only half of the truth. The way we react to stress appears to be more important than the stress itself."

Hans Selye, the world's foremost stress researcher, has stated that he believes no one can live without experiencing some degree of stress all the time. He believes that even the crossing of a busy intersection, exposure to a draft, or sheer joy is enough to activate the body's stress mechanisms to some extent. He also said that one's system must be prepared to handle stress and that the same stress that makes one person sick can create an invigorating experience for another.

When I talk to a new patient in my office, I always make sure I ask them these three questions:

1. What do you think is wrong with you?

2, How did you get this problem or pain?

3. Why do you have this problem?

I've found that all too often I hear "stress" as the answer to one or all of the questions.

"Dr. Gandee, I believe my daily headaches are caused by *stress* at my job."

"Dr. Gandee, I believe my stomach pain is caused by *stress* I am experiencing with my family."

"Dr. Gandee, I think my shoulder pain is just *stress-related*."

"Dr. Gandee, I'm sure my skin condition is caused by *stress* . . . the bills are piling up, and I don't know what to do."

Then I usually tell them that my job, working with sick and hurting people all day everyday is very stressful. We all seem to agree on that point. "I don't have headaches," I tell them. "So, if stress causes headaches, why don't I have headaches?" I also tell them I don't have stomach pain or shoulder pain, and they can look at my skin and see that it is rash-free. So it must be something else causing their problems.

It is true, however, that stress can set off an already weakened area of your body (a subluxated area). And a person under intense psychological stress is much more likely to have a weakened immune system. Stress can put more pressure on an already weakened system, but stress doesn't cause symptoms. If your body is strong in all areas, stress won't cause the symptoms many associate with it.

I always try to teach my patients that nerve interference is the bottom line. It is the basic reason for many symptoms. Sit-ting in a draft does not cause you to become sick; not wear-ing a hat doesn't cause you to become sick; and stress does not cause you to become sick, *if* your body is strong and in-terference-free to begin with. This is the key—the answer many people are seeking.

Some have argued that the absence of stress causes boredom. It is true that when there is "nothing going on," we do tend to get bored, some more quickly than others. If we can learn to handle, to manage, even to channel our stress, it can become a very positive force in our lives. It can mean a life of chal-lenge, excitement, and growth. There are even those who claim you cannot learn much without a certain amount of adversity—that "hard times" will make you a better, and certainly a stronger and wiser, person. This makes a lot of sense.

Countless famous people who write their autobiographies tell of intense personal despair and unrelenting stress that they en-countered in their lives, and they reveal that those were the times of their most notable accomplishments, creativity, insight, and personal growth. It is these "tests" of life that separate the survivors from those who simply give up on life.

How many copies of an autobiographical account do you think the public would buy if it were a simple story of some-one who had lived a very charmed life from the time he or she was a little baby, until he or she was a major success—all without any adverse episodes of any kind? Imagine a life with no ups and downs and no stress whatsoever. Boring? You bet. Best seller? No way! Would Scarlett O'Hara have been an in-teresting character if there had been no Civil War and no Rhett Butler, and she had just gone on living the easy life with good old never-rock-the-boat Ashley Wilkes at Tara? Fiddle-dee-dee, no, she wouldn't have been.

Stress is anything that upsets us or causes us to deviate from the path we thought we wanted to take. Stress means different things to different people. But the more positive your attitude, the better you'll handle stress, and the better your life will be.

I think that I have firmly established one very important fact. A depressed person has a depressed immune system. A happy person has a healthier immune system. This does not mean that miserable, unhappy people get sick and die, and all happy people go on forever skipping down the yellow brick road, but it does tell us that whatever you do and wherever you go, attitude *does* make a difference.

In 1982, two Harvard psychologists David McCelland and Carol Kirshnit did a study in which participants were made to watch a romantic movie under the researcher's assumption that a romantic movie would leave the participants feeling happy afterwards. The researchers noted that after watching the movie, the participants' levels of immunoglobulin-A ( one of the body's defenses against colds and other viral diseases) increased. Come on now, you gotta listen to results such as that.

Laughter and happiness hardly become bulletin news accounts on the 6 o'clock or 11 o'clock news, and they seldom show up in the bold headlines. But maybe they should!

## WHAT DOES ONE'S ATTITUDE HAVE TO DO WITH CHIROPRACTIC CARE?

The chiropractor has one goal in mind when you go to his or her office. He or she wants you to walk (and sometimes that's not easy) out of his or her office feeling better than when you came in. Any good chiropractor wants to make you healthy! Nothing gives me greater satisfaction than having my patients explain—often at length—just how much their lives have changed for the better after being under regular chiropractic care for a time. So, if we work together—the chiropractor on the adjustment of the spine, and the patients on the adjustment of their attitudes—chiropractic can turn the sickest and most pessimistic person into one you would hardly recognize.

It has been written that "no man is an island," and just as we cannot be totally separated from others; our bodies, minds, muscles, bones, nerves, and souls are all connected—one with another—and cannot be separated. This has been covered in Chapter 4. We are formed brain-first, then comes our spinal cord, to which all the rest is added and connected—all designed to work perfectly when aligned in the proper order. An adjustment of the spine will greatly improve your chances to keep your immune system working the way it was created to work, and if it works well, you will be in better health. If you are in better health, you will have a more positive attitude. Your outlook will be sunny, and your disposition will match it. Unlike the vicious cycle of a poorly working immune system making you feel worse, and feeling worse making your attitude worse; this chain of events is working in your favor. Your mental outlook mirrors your physical well-being.

## CHIROPRACTIC AND MENTAL HEALTH

Am I saying that chiropractic does away with mental illness and depression? No. But I will say that good health makes a difference in your entire system, and this includes your mental health. No one can make any guarantees, but I do believe that if more people were under chiropractic care, there would be a dramatic decrease in the number of mental illness patients in our country. Americans wouldn't be spending billions of dollars a year on antidepressant drugs, we would see a drop in suicides, and there would be less crime.

Oh, sure, you say, and the three little pigs would all live in brick houses, and nobody would cheat on their taxes. Am I a fool for believing this? I don't think so. Most will agree that a healthy, happy person makes better decisions, is a better citizen, cares more about his or her fellow Americans, and most important, is content and happy with him- or herself and those around him or her.

If we taught *real health* principles to our children, then we would start developing a society of healthier, better adjusted, well-nourished children. In an age where child-committed crime is soaring, we ought to be willing to consider all alternatives to correct this. Try to imagine a nation in which the children, as well as adults, toss away the junk food and nourish themselves with only healthy foods. Imagine our children getting daily exercise and having their spines checked to ensure that there is no interference in their wonderfully designed systems.

Your common sense should tell you that they would be much happier and healthier. There would be no need for mind-, mood-, or body-altering drugs. Their minds would be more pure because their bodies would be more pure. I'm not talking about a perfect world or perfect people or perfect anything for that matter, I'm talking about *making things better!* I'm talking about making life better for our children and for their children's children. I believe if we took some simple steps to teach our children well and to try to get them to do better than we have in taking care of ourselves, the world would certainly be a much better place.

- There would be less sickness.
- There would be less drug use.
- There would be less negativity.
- There would be less mental illness.
- There would be less crime.
- There would be less violence.
- There would be fewer premature deaths.
- Our children would be happier because they would be healthier.

Life, in general, would be better—much, much better.

It's not *what* happens to us but how we react to what happens to us that determines our lot in life—at least as far as health is concerned. It is the way we relate to people that dictates their reactions to us. The old pioneer searching for a new way of life with "good people" will find them because he left "good people" behind. Their attitudes were such that people responded nicely towards them. Hence these people were perceived as "good" people. The other family will find "mean-spirited and hateful people" wherever they go because that is what they left behind. If we looked at life in the same manner, we might be surprised to discover how much more positive and good our lives would be if we worked at it just a little more.

Those with a positive outlook and healthy attitude are many points ahead of the game at the starting bell. Even the statistic-crazed insurance companies have discovered that if a wife kisses her husband good-bye in the morning, he has fewer auto accidents and will live an average of five years longer. We have to believe this works in all aspects of life.

Attitude. Attitude. *Attitude.*

# Chapter 14

# Choices

*A little boy was overheard talking to himself as he walked through his backyard carrying his ball and bat. "I'm the greatest baseball player in the world," he said proudly. Then he tossed the ball in the air, swung at it, and missed.*

*Undaunted, he picked up the ball again, threw it into the air, and said to himself, "I'm the greatest player ever!" He missed the ball again.*

*He then paused for a moment to examine the bat and ball carefully. Then, with renewed vigor, he again threw the ball into the air and yelled, "I'm the greatest baseball player who ever lived." He swung the bat with much power and determination, and once again, he missed the elusive ball.*

*"Wow!" he exclaimed with some wonder. "What a great pitcher I am!"*

We may not be masters of our fate, but we do have choices to make in our lives. Sometimes the choices we make are verbalized, and sometimes they are only unspoken hopes and dreams. Other times we have to put our words and dreams into action in order to accomplish anything. Like the little boy with his baseball and bat, you must think about what it is that you are trying to accomplish, study that goal, and then *do it*. Then, we must look at what we are doing and decide if it is indeed the choice we wish to make.

"I don't care if my baby is a boy or a girl, as long as it's healthy."

Isn't this what you hear most often when you talk with expectant parents? Of course, it is. Most new mothers and fathers admit to checking the number of their new baby's fingers and toes and insuring that all the baby's body parts are intact upon that first inspection of this precious new being. Most people aren't overly concerned about the beauty of their child initially (although they are all beautiful). Our first concern centers around the health and well-being of this child, and we worry about his or her chances of remaining strong and healthy throughout life. We owe that to them, don't we?

What *else* do we owe them—and ourselves? What kind of a life would we offer our children if we insisted only that *they* be healthy, and we neglected our own health needs? It is just as important for a baby to have healthy parents as it is for a parent to have a healthy baby. In the child's early years, we are responsible for both.

If you have no children, then is it all right to abuse your health? You know it's not. You also know that you owe it to yourself to stay as healthy as possible. It's a choice you have to make. You argue the point by saying that heart disease and diabetes runs in your family, you were born with a defect; you've already suffered a debilitating disease; you have *no* choice. Wrong. You may have different choices than the man down the street, but you *always* have choices. Choices are closely tied to attitude, which we discussed in the previous chapter.

"But my doctor says I'll always be this way."

"I can't exercise . . . I'm too sick."

"I've always been puny. I was born that way, you can't change nature."

All of these excuses are just that—*excuses*. The best choice you can make for yourself today is to forget all those old excuses and begin your life anew, starting *right now*. Decide that you are going to be healthier and stronger, and life is going to be good to you because you are going to be good to yourself. Sounds simple doesn't it? Actually, it *is*. We often make simplicity complicated.

I could go even farther and ask how many of you have reached 100 percent or even 50 percent of your potential? No hands went up. Most of us do not live up to half of our potential. Is this the fault of your parents, your teachers, your spouse, your kids . . . yourself? I want you to take charge of your life—and your health. Let me ask one more question. How many of you are working at a job you hate? Some hands went up, didn't they? Are you continually living with a *wrong* choice?

## MY CHOSEN PROFESSION

I graduated from the University of Akron (Ohio) in 1976 with a degree in education and a minor in health. I thought I wanted to be a teacher until I got into the classroom. It turned out that teaching wasn't what I expected it to be at all. It seemed like the attitude of the students was all wrong—or maybe it was my attitude that was wrong.

My reasons for wanting to be a teacher were the right ones. I wanted to help shape and direct young people's minds. I truly believed then—and I still do—that my first goal was a worthy one. I was devastated when the realization hit me that I did not like teaching. Fortunately, I was only a student teacher at the time, but it was clear to me as soon as I went into the classroom that this was not for me. I was both amazed and discouraged when I took note of the basic changes in our education system. The kids were different. The teachers were different. Times were different from when I was in school. Most of all, I was different.

It was a terrible time for me. There I was, soon to be a college graduate, ready to assume my place in life, ready to accept major responsibility, and I found out that my chosen occupation for which I'd gone to school for four years was something I didn't like—*not even a little bit*. What on earth was I going to do?

I could have stuck it out. I could have hoped things would get better, that in time I would be a good teacher and the students would learn something from me. I still believe teaching is one of the most honorable professions in the world. But for teachers who do not enjoy teaching, it has to be absolute misery for both them and the students. I did myself—and the students I would have tried to teach—a big favor by admitting my mistake, then and there.

Do you think it was easy for me to do this? Absolutely not! My first thought was that I had wasted four years of my life to learn an occupation that I could not imagine working in for the rest of my life. I had made my choices for all the right reasons, and it had turned out to be all wrong.

Did I learn from this mistake? Of course, I did. I must confess, I chose my next profession for all the wrong reasons, but it turned out to be the right choice. I can honestly tell you that I now love what I do. And strangely enough, I am still a teacher. I'm just teaching different things to different people. There is, however, a confession I must make. When I went to chiropractic school, one of my strongest motivations was a financial one. I thought chiropractors made a lot of money, and since I was going to have to go back to school, I certainly needed a lot of money. I wasn't thrilled with the fact that I was now facing four more *long* years of school. In addition to that, I was concerned about how intense and demanding the education requirements for chiropractic were. So, basically, I had a little talk with myself about it.

"Give it your best shot," I told myself. "Put the time, effort, and energy into the schooling and offer no excuses when it's over and done." I was content with the choice I had made. In time (but certainly not right away), I would know for a fact that it was the absolute right choice.

I started chiropractic school in Marietta, Georgia in the month of July. If you've ever been to Georgia in July, and you have any problems at all with allergies or hay fever like I did, then I don't have to tell you how hot and miserable I was. So, there I was in school *(again)*, eyes red and swollen, nose running, coughing and choking, and just trying to breathe and see. It was more than difficult to listen to anything the instructor was saying. I was, to put it simply, a real mess.

As I sat in class from 8:00 a.m. until 4:00 p.m., five days a week, I heard about how chiropractic was not only good for backaches, whiplashes, and strains. Through the haze of nose sprays and allergy medication, I began to hear how chiropractic had helped many varied health problems from headaches and ulcers to asthma and sciatica. Then one day a professor mentioned something about how effective chiropractic was with allergies. Allergies!

He certainly got my attention with that statement. I almost went through the roof. There I was, still suffering miserably with every terrible allergy symptom known to humankind, and this guy was standing up in front of the class saying that chiropractic could help my allergies. What drivel, I thought.

By this time a few weeks had passed, and I had received a couple of chiropractic adjustments from student clinicians. However, my allergy symptoms still persisted, of course. I couldn't believe what that man was saying. I admitted that I might be mercenary for going into a profession because I thought I could make a lot of money, but, hey, I had ethics, and I did draw the line at this kind of thing. I knew I could not be a part of this nonsense. I decided I would not, or *could* not, be a chiropractor and claim that I could help these conditions if chiropractic didn't help me.

Fuming in my seat, I shook my overstuffed head and clenched my teeth together to keep from jumping up in class and telling everybody what a big bunch of baloney all this was. It was total misrepresentation, I thought. It was, in clear terms, a boldfaced lie, and I wasn't going to go along with it.

I left the class and went immediately to see Dr. Charlie Kalb, D.C., the vice president of academic affairs at the college. "I'm quitting," I said, even before I sat down in the chair across from his desk. He asked me why. "Because they're *lying*," I answered bluntly. By this time I was really on the edge. My allergy-ridden anger was kicking in. My voice was rising. My face was contorted, and my vision was clouded.

Dr. Kalb looked me straight in the eye and said in a very calm voice, "Tell me about it." I would remember those four words again and again in my life and realize they were probably right up at the top of the list of most important words, such as "I love you" and "the check is in the mail."

So I told him about it. And he listened. When Dr. Kalb said "tell me about it," I could tell he was genuinely interested in what I was saying and feeling at the time.

"They're *lying* to us in the classroom," I repeated. "The instructor said chiropractic can help people with all types of health problems, including allergy sufferers. Well, just look at me. I'm miserable. It's a *lie!* I went on to tell him that I might do a lot of things to make money, but I was not going into a profession where out-and-out fraud was practiced. "Why did he say that people with these problems can be helped by chiropractic when they can't?" I asked the man seated across the desk from me.

"They *can* be helped," Dr. Kalb said, his voice extremely calm. I glared at him.

"If the allergy is related to the spinal nerve impingement or subluxation, then we can be of great help to the patient," he explained.

"But look at *me!*" I was almost yelling by this time, as I offered myself as a prime example—red-eyed, runny nose, and all. "I'm telling you, it didn't help me at all, and I've been getting adjustments."

Prior to chiropractic school, I'd only gone to a chiropractor once. I was 21 years old at the time. Early one Sunday morning, I had sneezed and threw my back out. I couldn't believe that such a simple thing could cause so much pain. I went to my family doctor because I could not breathe. I was in severe pain and suffering from spasms that would knock me to my knees. In addition, I was really scared. Nothing like that had ever happened to me before.

Immediately, I was put on drugs and given heat therapy. But that didn't help. The pain was still there, and I was getting very little sleep. I was told it would take time, so I toughed it out for a couple of months. Finally, someone mentioned the option of chiropractic care to me. I had to admit that I'd never even heard of a chiropractor before and had little confidence in something so foreign to me. Pain ruled, however, and I finally called for an appointment.

He was one of those old-time chiropractors with no assistants, no staff, no x-rays—just him and his hands. When I went into his office, I was very apprehensive about getting on the table. I must say, he really worked me over, doing several adjustments to my spine. It didn't hurt, although I thought it would since I was already in such pain, but it was all very different from anything I'd ever experienced before.

He was also a man of few words, and even though I wanted to ask questions, I didn't, and he certainly didn't take the time to explain anything to me. "That'll be $9.00," he said when he was finished.

I gave him the money, and he stuffed it down in his pocket and dismissed me. To tell the truth, I felt as though I'd just been ripped off for the nine bucks. When I got back home, I was so tired that I went to bed immediately and fell into a deep sleep for five hours. When I woke up, I was somewhat surprised that I felt better. I wasn't 100-percent better. I'd been hurting too long to have achieved that kind of recovery, but I was certainly improved and didn't feel nearly so resentful about handing over my money to the old man. I had no idea why or how his treatment helped me, but I still remembered that old doctor that day in Georgia as I sat across from Dr. Kalb.

"Tell me about your medical care for allergies," Dr. Kalb said, bringing me back to the present.

"Well, Dr. Kalb, when I was five or six years old, my mother took me to the Cleveland Clinic, where I was given a battery of shots to determine the source of my allergies," I said. "I remember ten to fifteen shots in each arm with a needle stuck just under skin." I also added that it hurt. I remembered crying very hard, but they told me it had to be done so they could find out exactly what I was allergic to, so they could help me get better. After the tests, they told my mother what I was allergic to and gave us a prescription. I started going to my family doctor three times weekly for shots. I did this for about ten years, in addition to taking a prescription for medication that I was still taking when I entered chiropractic college. I reached into my pocket and pulled out the pills I'd been living on all those years and showed them to Dr. Kalb, who looked at them without comment.

"How long did you say you've been under chiropractic care?" he asked.

"I'm a mess," I said, not really answering his question.

"How long have you been getting adjustments?" he asked again, still trying to get a straight answer out of me.

"I had one in Akron about four years ago, and I've had two since I've been in Georgia. Again, I just wish you'd look at what a mess I'm in. Do I look like a well person to you?" By this time I was more angry than ever. I punctuated my argument with a deep sniffle and a dry cough.

He laughed, which made me even madder. He laughed harder. I was out of my chair by this time, and repeating my serious threat to leave school. I would not deal with their lies, and I certainly would not perpetuate them by joining the ranks of misrepresenters. This was not a choice I was having any difficulty with at all! I was gone!

"Sit down, sit down," Dr. Kalb said, waving his hand in my direction. "Now, let's see if I have this right . . ." he leaned back in his chair and repeated my allergy history. "When you were five years old, you were taken to the Cleveland Clinic where you received a series of shots and remained on them three times a week for the next ten years."

I nodded. He had been listening well.

"You've continued with some form of traditional medicine, even up until this time?"

I nodded again.

"Let's see," he said, closing his eyes to count. "That makes about twenty-one years you've had the shots and medicine. You've given them a lot of time to help your problems, but it's obvious that you still suffer a great deal."

Again I nodded vigorously, between coughing and wiping my raw, red eyes.

"And you've had *three* chiropractic adjustments in your lifetime that have also failed to correct the problem. Is that right?"

Right. It was beginning to become clear to me. I had done what most people have done—stayed in a situation where medicine wasn't helping much, yet I failed to seek alternatives.

"I don't want you to forget what has happened here today," Dr. Kalb said then. "In the coming years, some of your patients are going to act and feel the same way you have felt today. And because they will be suffering and will not feel they are being helped, they will find it difficult, if not impossible, to understand." He paused for a moment, then leaned across the desk. "How many times did you or your parents ever say to your medical doctor, 'Hey, doc, my son has gotten three shots a week for five to ten years . . . yet he's *still* sick. Why? Why not just one shot to heal him? Why not just one pill to stop his problems? Why all this treatment, and yet he still suffers? What kind of a profession do you have?' Were those questions ever asked?"

"We never asked," I replied, rather stunned at my own revelation.

"That's what I thought," he said. "Most people say very little, if anything, to their medical doctors. They just take the medication for years, as they keep on suffering. They are still sick and still in pain. In many cases they are referred to another doctor or doctors, and he or she proceeds to put them to sleep and cut them open, still with very few questions."

It was like the dawning of a new morning for me. My eyes were opening, still red and watery at this point, but I was starting to understand this thing called chiropractic. In time, I would come to appreciate it more than I could have believed possible.

Dr. Kalb went further as I sat in his office. He explained that most people have no problem at all asking pointed questions to a chiropractor, becoming extremely critical and often rude at times. He used, as an example, my anger at chiropractic, the school, and even at him.

"Here you are, ready to quit school because you are not healed after just two adjustments," he said. "You've given medicine years and years to do the job, and it hasn't. You don't seem angry at the medical profession, yet you blame us for not making you well with two or three adjustments. Does any of this make sense to you?"

Almost meekly then, I asked him what he thought I should do—choices again.

"Stay in school, and *listen* to what we're saying and *why* we're saying it," he replied. "Then see for yourself how a variety of people with different illnesses come to the school clinic for help. Check their results and keep your mind open to change and to new ways of treating various illnesses. No one profession has all the answers, but I think you'll be amazed at the truly remarkable ability the body has to heal itself—which is what chiropractic is all about."

I felt rather chagrined. "I don't suppose there has been quite enough time for me to feel the effects of my chiropractic treatments for my allergies," I said, much quieter at this point than when I first walked into his office.

"Not quite," Dr. Kalb said, smiling. "All I ask is that you give the school and chiropractic a chance. You deserve it, and so does the rest of the world, especially your future patients. I think you understand what I'm saying."

I did. And it was just the beginning of my understanding. My understanding was further underscored the following year by the fact that I was able to get through the allergy season with much more ease and comfort. I was getting regular adjustments, and by the end of the year I no longer had to rely on the medication I'd used for so long. My body was beginning to heal itself. I have never again had to take medication to control my allergies—and thanks to chiropractic care, my allergies no longer control me.

## THE LESSONS I'VE LEARNED

One important thing that I learned from that experience is the importance of the art of listening. If you ask a person a question, listen to the answer. I can always tell if a person is truly listening to what it is that I have to say. One's body language says it all. Listening shows interest, respect, caring, and love. Now, when my patients come into my office and tell me that things are not going well, I never dismiss their complaints. I always ask them to tell me about it, and I listen.

Not all of our education is gained in the classroom. This is especially true when it comes to our own good health. We need to educate ourselves because no one else will do it for us. I conduct health talks in my office regularly. It is a prerequisite for my new patients to attend at least one of these lectures. I talk about my philosophy of health, in general, and chiropractic, in particular.

In all the years that I've been giving these health talks, No one has ever told me that they didn't like what they heard— not even once. Everyone who has attended tells me they have learned more about their own health and that they leave with a much better understanding of their own bodies. I try to give them enough information about their own good health in hope that they will want to learn more and continue to practice these principles.

At a recent meeting, which also included some other chiropractors—as some of my meetings do—one of my patients got up and gave a marvelous speech about how much he and his family had been helped by chiropractic care over the years. He thanked the chiropractic profession profusely and expressed his absolute gratitude to us. In conclusion, he very calmly and thoroughly let the members of the chiropractic profession have it with both barrels.

"I want to admonish you because we are having an absolute crisis in health care," he said, and we all knew he was not speaking about some governmental health-care plan up for a vote.

"I don't care what the title of your practice is," he continued. "I don't care what initials follow your name. I don't care what colleges you went to—I just want to tell you that there is a desperate health crisis in the United States, and we haven't heard or seen nearly enough from you folks—the chiropractors."

I squirmed uneasily because I knew he was right. I looked around me, and I could tell the others were feeling the discomfort as well.

"I haven't seen enough of you on television—I see medical doctors all the time. I haven't seen enough of you writing letters to the editors—I see letters from medical doctors almost every week. I haven't seen enough popular press articles written by or about chiropractors. I always see a medical doctor's by-line. When I say 'I'm going to the chiropractor,' some people say, 'Oh, no, not me. No way,' and what do they *really know* about chiropractors? Nothing, except what they've been fed by the medical profession." He was just getting warmed up. There was more—much more.

"They have not heard from you," he continued, his voice rising as he spoke. "And I chastise you for not taking a more aggressive stance. I realize you have been attacked for generations by the American Medical Association, and I can understand your reluctance to take on a Goliath of this nature, but it can—and it *must*—be done!"

He also asked us if we didn't do it, *who* would? We all knew the answer—nobody! He was absolutely right. It's time we as chiropractors and as caring human beings stood up—and we can stand up straight—and allow ourselves to be counted before we're counted out! Silence is acceptance.

I know that some chiropractors still fear the consequences of speaking out. Many still remember the time when chiropractors were imprisoned for practicing their profession. However, this is the type of history chiropractic has to overcome. With this kind of condemnation, the profession was almost prevented

# Did You Know...

... that the British Research Council on Complementary Medicine diligently sought to find proof of the effectiveness of alternative medicine, which they defined as long-standing and well-structured therapies, such as acupuncture, chiropractic, homeopathy, medical herbalism, naturopathy, osteopathy, and some of the newer relaxation techniques, such as biofeedback and dietary programs. Much of the open-minded attitude of those on the council can be attributed to Prince Charles, who suggested in a speech that doctors in England give serious consideration to alternative methods of treatment.

from telling the story. Chiropractors just did their jobs quietly and kept their mouths shut out of fear of reprisal. It doesn't matter that as a profession we have been greatly misrepresented and ridiculed. It doesn't matter that we receive less respect than we deserve. As dedicated health-care professionals, we must tell the story now, regardless of any fear of consequences. I am very pleased to see that more and more chiropractors are getting more and more courageous and much more willing to spread the word about the wonder of our profession. We *must* share our knowledge of *the better way*—and just as important, we must eradicate *The Big Lie*!

For years there has been a concentrated and deliberate effort on the part of organized medicine headed up by the AMA and eleven other medical organizations, to suppress and eliminate the entire profession of chiropractic. Am I just being paranoid? No, this is a fact.

## THE LESSONS THAT I HOPE YOU HAVE LEARNED

By the time you reach this part of the book, I hope you are extremely aware of the importance of your mind-body connection and realize that you do have a voice as far as your own well-being is concerned. I cannot emphasize the following phrase enough: *It's up to you!*

If you smoke, follow a poor diet, drink to excess, or are over-weight, your life might continue in the same way it always has, at least for awhile. However, fate has a way of handing us sur-prises now and then. Sometimes the surprise is not pleasant. It should frighten any of us to discover that more than half of the time, one of the first signs of a heart attack is *death*. Now, if that is not a basic fact for us to face, I don't know what is. Death offers us no second chances. With death there is no chance to change our eating habits, reduce stress, revise our lifestyles, exercise—nothing. It's over and done. Boom! You're dead. We cannot back up and say to ourselves that we will be more careful from now on. That ship's done sailed.

Americans have been conditioned to believe that no symp-toms means no sickness, no symptoms means no disease, and no symptoms means good health. In chiropractic, we have a saying: "Symptoms are the first to leave, and the last to ap-pear." What that means is that once a dis-ease process sets up in your body, it takes time, sometimes years, before we actual-ly realize we have a problem (hence, *the last to appear*).

Let's say you own an old farm way back in the country, and you seldom get the chance to visit the old abandoned house. If someone came and took up residence in the house, you wouldn't know it unless you saw it for yourself or someone told you. Once you found it out, it was evident to you that you had a problem. Symptoms are the message we receive that something is amiss, and until we find out, or are informed that there is a problem, we are completely in the dark. The squat-ter could be ruining what was left of your old house, and you would not be aware of it until it was too late.

The same thing happens when there is disease in the body. The body didn't want to bother you at first with something it may have been able to handle itself. It fights a valiant battle every second of every hour to ward off disease, but sometimes the problem becomes more than the body can handle, especially if we aren't helping the body by living a careless lifestyle. When the body weakens to the point that it begins to give off symp-toms, the illness may very well have a firm grip on you. One of the most common symptoms is pain. The body is saying, "Hey, I fought a good fight. I've tried for years to keep this thing contained. I've worked my little hiney off fighting this thing for you, but it's getting the best of me, and I need your help. I can't handle this by myself any longer." Pain is the alarm, the wake-up call. Pain lets us know something is wrong. And, unlike the man whose pain was a heart attack that killed him, you, at least, have a second chance to make some very important choices.

One of your choices would be to stop the pain. Wouldn't that help? It would, of course, if the pain were unbearable, and sometimes it is. But, basically, when people make the choice of taking a painkiller, they are merely ridding themselves of the alarm. They believe that by getting rid of the pain, they have eliminated the cause as well. Ask yourself, if the pain is gone, is my illness gone as well? Unfortunately, that is not the case.

Take the scenario of the man who was sleeping soundly when his fire alarm went off. It was a terrible sound that woke him from his sleep and scared the daylights out of him. His heart was pounding as he jumped out of bed. Looking at his watch, he realized that he was late for work. He didn't have time to check on any stupid alarm. So, what did he do? He simply yanked the batteries out to stop the annoying noise, threw on his clothes, and went to work.

Was he smart? Was it a false alarm, or did he come home that night to discover only ashes? His only concern was getting rid of the noise. He didn't care *why* the alarm was sounding, only that it was, and he put a stop to it. By stopping the alarm, did he solve his problem? Is he safe now that the alarm is off? Of course not.

It is the same story when we get rid of our pain with a pill. The pain may be relieved, at least for a time, but if there is a serious reason for it, it will return—if you're lucky. Then, again, your choice to make will be what to do about it. Most people know, whether they act upon it or not, that masking or hiding the pain is putting off the inevitable. It is a choice that could have fatal consequences.

You have noticed by now, I'm sure, that I tend to harp on some subjects. I do repeat myself because I want to make sure that you understand what I am saying. The truth always bears repeating, and you can never hear it too much. I recall an English teacher I once had who was trying to teach us meanings of various words. The word "repetition" was on the list, and when she got to it, she asked the squirming fourth-graders if anyone knew what the word meant. No hands went up. She looked around the room, then slowly began to repeat the word: *repetition, repetition, repetition, repetition,* until I would venture to say that there is not one child in that class who will not remember for the rest of his or her life what "repetition" means.

So, when it comes to masking pain, I cannot repeat too much that it is a dangerous practice. I will point out here that I am not against taking something to alleviate certain kinds of pain, but we must not use that as a "cure" because it is not. We can continue suffering for a long time in some cases, and we can sometimes kill the pain depending on the cause. Or we can make some other choices.

We could see a chiropractor. Oh sure, you say, Dr. Gandee is being self-serving here. Of course, I am. At the same time I am also serving *your* self. You have no idea how much satisfaction I get from having a patient come in with pain that I can ease without painkillers or surgery. I am looking at, and treating, the *cause* of the pain, and it doesn't take an Einstein to figure out that once the *cause* of the pain is gone—so is the pain.

When a patient comes to me with pain, I do the standard tests and x-rays. Often I find a misaligned vertebra that is causing nerve interference, and, in turn, causing the pain. I suggest a program of chiropractic care and sometimes simple exercises to fix the problem. I may suggest a treatment three times a week until positive changes in the structure of the spine are apparent. And guess what happens. The biggest problem in chiropractic health care occurs. *It works.* After a few treatments, the patient's symptoms begin to lessen, and often disappear completely.

"Aha," the patients think. "I'm cured . . . no more pain." Now they have choices to make again. "No point in going to the chiropractor anymore," they decide. "If there is no more pain, there is no point in putting out good money. I feel fine!"

The pain may be gone, but the patient is not healed—not yet. He or she may be well on his or her way, but since there is no more pain, he or she feels as though everything is fine. Everything is not. It was not fine *before* the pain, either, and the disease continues to do damage to his or her body. The adjustments have helped the body to the point where it is "handling things" again, but sometimes the problem is not solved.

It is at this point in chiropractic care that many patients make that very unwise choice. They decide to stop going to the chiropractor. They no longer have to follow his or her instructions. The pain is gone, the tingling is better, the ache is tolerable. Chiropractic has done the job. They are healed. There is no point in continuing this. That doctor just wants their money.

The truth is that the chiropractor understands the way the body works. We try (and too often fail) to educate our patients about this very critical point. We try to tell them that just because they feel well (which is wonderful) and the pain has subsided (such relief) that they may not be healed. I wish they were absolutely well once the pain disappears, but that is not always so. Again, I repeat to you, in order to be healthy, you must *work at being healthy*—and this includes regular chiropractic checkups and care.

The body wants very much to be healthy. It constantly strives to be healthy by continually working, improving, changing itself to be fit. The bottom line is that the body really does *talk* (sometimes it even yells) to us. The next important thing is that we have got to learn to *listen* to it. You are responsible for your own good health. Not your family, your friends, your medical doctor, your dog, your minister, your barber, or your fortune teller. *You* are responsible!

I am astonished at how often patients come into my office in real pain without a clue to how the pain came about. They say that they woke up that morning with terrible pain for no reason at all, and they can't imagine what caused it. It is at this point that I start thinking that this is likely a symptom of some old injury they suffered years ago but was never fixed. They took an aspirin for the pain—maybe something stronger—and it went away. It was "cured." They may have had a car accident that "didn't amount to anything," fallen out of a tree when they were a kid (all kids do, nothing to it), stumbled on a flight of stairs, tripped, slipped on ice, lifted something too heavy—any number of things.

"Oh, that—that was nothing—it happened years ago. It's over and done with." Don't bet on it. The body has fought off that old injury for years, but now it's time to pay the piper.

Here's an example. When Tina was 16 years old, she was riding in a car when it was hit from behind. Her neck was sore for a few days, but she was OK. She was never checked by a chiropractor or a medical doctor because it was just no big deal. She took a few aspirin and had some good bed rest, she skipped a couple of days school, and life was as good as ever. She's 34 now and under my care. She has numbing pain in her left arm, pain in her shoulders, stiffness in her neck, and she complains of daily headaches—has had them for years, she says. Yes, she has been to medical doctors. Some of them made her feel as though it was "all in her head," and at times she begins to think that maybe they're right. A pill here and there brought her some relief, but the problem was still there—and getting worse.

The x-rays show that her neck lacked a proper curve, a disc in her spine was beginning to deteriorate (usually due to old injury, often forgotten) and she had some misaligned vertebrae (which could also be due to old injury). These were not new problems for this patient. She had lived with it for years hoping it would "cure" itself, but it had only gotten worse, instead of better. She made the choice to ignore the problem, but the problem decided it no longer wants to be ignored.

When I suggested that this condition stemmed from an old injury from years ago, she had to search her brain to recall any such accident. Many patients often do not even remember anything that would have caused problems, but somewhere in their past something did happen to cause a subluxation, which in turn, later caused numerous and sometimes extremely serious problems.

When this patient had the accident, she was young and healthy, and her immune system was in good working order. Her body was able to fight its own battles and continued to do so with few symptoms for several years. When the numbness in the arm, the shoulder pain, and the other discomforts started, she became alarmed. The body was telling her that it had had enough of fighting alone, and now she has to seek help to help her body get well again.

Tina began undergoing regular chiropractic treatments, and we were able to correct those problems that were causing so many problems for her. She is much more aware of the way her body operates now. It is satisfying to be able to alleviate her pain for the present, and to assure her that this particular problem, if checked periodically, should not cause her further pain or discomfort. Even more important, it will not develop into something that cannot be corrected.

There are four stages of illness. What I want my patients to know is that when they are feeling ill or in pain, they are experiencing what I call the *third* stage of illness or dis-ease. They are not happy when I tell them what the *fourth* stage is . . .

The four stages are:

1. *The Cause*—Interference to the life expression. It is whatever is responsible for the beginning of your health problem.

2. *The Condition*—If you don't heal yourself of the *cause*, then you have a *condition*. This is brought about by the prolonged presence of the *cause*. Although your body can often handle itself for awhile, with time, the *condition* gets worse until you reach the third stage.

3. *Symptoms*—When you finally have *symptoms*, and when you realize that something is wrong, you become aware of the *condition* and need to search for the *cause*.

4. *Death*—The state in which your body can no longer fight off the *cause* of its *symptoms*.

When patients realize that the symptom stage comes right before the death stage, their attention is piqued. When I explain that standard medical treatment works directly with the third stage of disease, rather than treating the cause, they are even more alert. As a doctor of chiropractic, I realize that the absence of symptoms does not necessarily mean the presence of health. The patient can be at the first or second stage of disease and be totally unaware of it. Only after the first stage, the *cause,* is removed, can health be fully restored.

Nobody can convince you that you feel better when you do not. It is my sincere hope that this book will help open more eyes to the fact that there is so much more to health care than popping a pill, submitting to the knife, or living in constant pain without hope. By now I believe you know there is *a better way.*

We don't always choose the better way. Sometimes we have accepted certain ideas as fact for so long that it is difficult to see the forest clearly because of the trees. I meet patients with all kinds of preconceived notions and opinions. I try to listen to them, in hopes they might also listen to me. I can understand how the general public has come to almost revere our medical doctors.

All of chiropractic's case histories are not "happily-ever-after" stories. I recall one particular patient, an elderly man, who came to my office in considerable pain. He filled out the normal case history form and was led into the consultation room by a member of my staff.

When I entered the room, I could immediately sense that working with him was not going to be a piece of cake. To say that he was going to be a very difficult patient would have been kind. He looked rather uncomfortable and was seated on the edge of a chair, strumming his fingers defiantly. I glanced at his history form, which told me he was suffering from very painful sciatica that worsened at night. He also had problems with urination—he would begin urinating, maintaining a stream; but then his urine would begin dribbling, and he could not completely void the bladder. These are some of the possible symptoms of prostate cancer. I had no way of knowing if he was aware of this, and if he were aware, I wondered if this was the cause of his obvious agitation.

I asked a few questions. He gave me curt and clipped answers. It was easy to see that the man neither liked nor trusted me. Furthermore, it would appear that he had no intention of changing his mind. I wondered why he had come to me in the first place. Actually, he did not come in *the first place*. As is often the case with many chiropractic patients, chiropractic was his *last* resort, and he had little confidence that anything would work at this point.

I asked a few more questions, and he continued to be totally obstinate. Finally I said, "Sir, you act as if you don't like me."

"I don't *know* you," he answered sharply. "I don't know you, don't trust you." Well, he certainly didn't beat around the bush.

"Why is that?" I asked, trying to be as diplomatic as I could.

"Because you're a *doctor*, that's why."

"But you came to me . . . "

"I've been to lots of other doctors," he snapped. "They cost me lots of money, I've taken lots of drugs, been through lots of test. I still hurt, and I don't trust doctors anymore."

"But still you came to me today," I repeated.

"I heard you were good," he growled, almost under his breath.

"But you don't believe it," I finished for him.

He glared at me without answering.

"I'd like to do an x-ray of your lower back," I said then, trying to ignore the open hostility. "Then I want to do a few orthopedic tests."

"Nope." The reply was short and anything but sweet.

I smiled at him and asked if he would repeat his answer.

"Nope," he said again, his frown deepening. "No x-rays, no tests. I'm here for a chiropractic adjustment. I heard you are good at that, and that's what I want done. No more. No less. I'm giving you *one* chance, and that's it." I seldom get offered an ultimatum like that.

"Are you serious, sir," I asked, looking closely at the crotchety old man.

"I am," he said without hesitation. "One chance, and that's it. Fix me or not. It's up to you." Well, at least he gave me a choice.

I sat down so that we were on the same eye level and looked directly at him. "Do I understand that you've had this problem for a long time?"

"Two-and-a-half years," he replied without blinking.

"You've had this problem for a period of two-and-a-half years, and you've been to numerous doctors, been through batteries of tests, taken bottles of medication, had physical therapy over a period of several months, and nothing has helped?" I asked, glancing at his history again.

"That's right," he said, looking me straight in the eye.

"And you are limiting me to *one* adjustment, *one* treatment. Is that correct?" I asked him, just to make sure I'd heard him right. Remember to *listen to the patient,* I told myself.

"Yes, that's correct," he said, folding his arms across his chest and jutting his chin forward. "One adjustment. You're *supposed* to be good. Fix me."

Very slowly, I put his chart down on the chair and looked at him for a few moments before speaking. Finally, I told him in the calmest manner that I could that I would accept him as a patient for this one treatment. "But it's going to cost you $100,000," I added.

He almost had a heart attack. When he finally regained his composure and his ability to speak, he spat out the words in anger and disbelief. "$100,000 for *one* adjustment!!! Are you absolutely *nuts?*"

"No," I told him as kindly as I could. "You didn't come here for treatment. You are here for *a miracle,* and if I do miracles, I have to charge miracle prices."

Although I had no idea what the market price of miracles was that day, I knew they couldn't be cheap. Needless to say, he made the decision to decline my "miracle" price. You can't win 'em all. With some, you can't even get into the game.

I will admit that sometimes it is discouraging when patients fail to heed my advice—and I know realistically that it will continue to happen. Another one of the reasons I wrote this book is so my patients (and the general public) can read the printed word and (I hope) refer to it from time to time, until they are fully educated and convinced about the ways chiropractic care really works. I want you to understand exactly what it can mean to a person. It is often the difference between a good healthy life, and one that is pain-ridden and full of despair.

It's a simple choice, really, but many fail to grasp the full impact of what this choice can mean to them and their families. One thing I do know, even though I work extremely hard trying to explain to each and every one of my patients how the body works, why the body hurts, how they can help themselves now, and what they can do to make their health better in the future, the vast majority of them are *not* going to do what I suggest. They may trust me as a doctor and even like me as a person, but life is too intense, too hectic, too busy, and too stressful, so they will just throw up their hands and say, "Oh well, Dr. Gandee means well, but I can't do all these things."

They will receive only symptomatic care, and I am sure they *will* be back. It may be in three months, a year, or even five years, but if they left soon after the cessation of their symptoms, then they will return, just as the symptoms will. They will come into the office with the same problems as before. They will tell me the same stories and offer the same complaints. I will, in turn, tell them the same story of health I told them before, the *real* story of health that chiropractors have been telling for 100 years.

It is my earnest hope that you will continue to study and learn about chiropractic care, then utilize it in your life. I hope you make the right choice of trying chiropractic and giving it a chance to prove that it works in harmony with your body to offer you overall health benefits. I know without a shadow of a doubt that if chiropractic care were to become part of mainstream health care, it would revolutionize the system as we know it, and it would offer us a country—and even a world —of much healthier and happier individuals. With chiropractic care, you can triumph over illness.

Is that fantasy? Could it happen? I think it could. The bottom line is that it all comes down to choice—your choice. You are the *only* one who can make the difference. Chiropractors can't—and shouldn't—make the choice for you. The medical profession can't—and shouldn't—make the choice for you. We still live in a free country of choices, and if you can find a better way to get something done to insure your good health, then do it.

You are the only one who can choose what kind of health you will have for the rest of your life. And even though I can't tell you what to do, I can perhaps nudge, even push sometimes, in the direction of naturally good health.

Let's hope you never find yourself having to make a choice between facing a jungle full of wild animals and swimming across a stream filled with snakes and alligators. But just in case that ever does happen, it would be best if you were in the *best* possible condition!

When I say there is a better way, what I really mean is that there is a healthier way, and you are in the driver's seat. I can put up road signs and directions. I can offer maps and pointers, and I can even write a book offering advice about which turn you should make and which direction you should consider—but in the end, the story is still the same. The road you take is *your choice.*

If you enjoyed this book and found it to be helpful, you have any comments or additional questions about how alternative health care can improve your quality of life, you would like help in finding a good chiropractor in your area, or you would like to have Dr. Gandee speak to your organization, you may contact him by telephone: 1-800-724-6435, e-mail: info@drgandee .com, or via the internet: http://www.drgandee.com.

# Suggested Readings

Franks, Richard A. *Prepare for Success*. Athens, GA: Agee Publishers, Inc., 1992. 1-800-775-7900

James, Walene. *Immunization: The Reality Behind the Myth*. Connecticut: Bergin and Garvey Publishers, Inc., 1995.

McKenna, John. *Alternatives to Antibiotics*. Garden City Park, NY: Avery Publishing Group, 1998.

Mendelsohn, Robert S. *Confessions of a Medical Heretic*. Chicago: Contemporary Books, 1990.

Schmidt, Michael A., Smith, Lendon H., Sehnert, Keith W. *Beyond Antibiotics: Boost Your Immunity and Avoid Antibiotics*. Berkelely: North Atlantic Books, 1994.

Strauss, Joseph B. *Enhance Your Life Experience*. Levittown, PA: Foundation for Advancement of Chiropractic Education, 1996. 1-800-397-9722

Wilk, Chester A. *Medicine, Monopolies, and Malice: How the Medical Establishment Tried to Destroy Chiropractic in the U.S.* Garden City Park, NY: Avery Publishing Group, 1996.

# Index

# Healthy Habits
## *are easy to come by—*
## If You Know Where to Look!

## To get the latest information on:
- better health • diet & weight loss
- the latest nutritional supplements
- herbal healing & homeopathy and more

**COMPLETE AND RETURN THIS CARD RIGHT AWAY!**

Where did you purchase this book?

❑ bookstore     ❑ health food store     ❑ pharmacy

❑ supermarket     ❑ other (please specify)_____

Name _____

Street Address _____

City _____ State _____ Zip _____

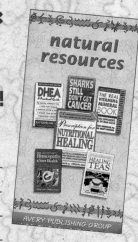

# Trying to eat healthier? Looking to lose weight? Frustrated with bland-tasting fat-free foods?

For more information on how you can create low-fat meals that are packed with taste and nutrition and develop healthy habits that can improve the quality of your life,

**COMPLETE AND RETURN THIS CARD!**

Where did you purchase this book?

❑ bookstore     ❑ health food store     ❑ pharmacy

❑ supermarket     ❑ other (please specify)_____

Name _____

Street Address _____

City _____ State _____ Zip _____

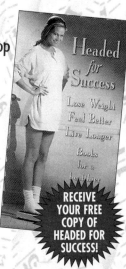

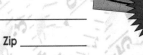

RECEIVE YOUR FREE COPY OF HEADED FOR SUCCESS!

PLACE
STAMP
HERE

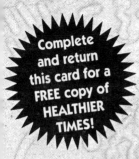
Complete
and return
this card for a
FREE copy of
HEALTHIER
TIMES!

## AVERY PUBLISHING GROUP
### 120 Old Broadway
### Garden City Park, NY 11040

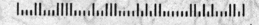

PLACE
STAMP
HERE

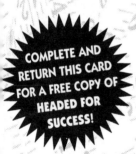
COMPLETE AND
RETURN THIS CARD
FOR A FREE COPY OF
HEADED FOR
SUCCESS!

## AVERY PUBLISHING GROUP
### 120 Old Broadway
### Garden City Park, NY 11040